Good Days, Bad Days

Good Days, Bad Days

The Self in Chronic Illness and Time

Kathy Charmaz

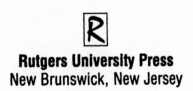

Rutgers University Press
New Brunswick, New Jersey

The following publishers have given permission to quote from copyrighted works: From *Episode: Report on the Accident Inside My Skull*, by Eric Hodgins. © 1963 by Eric Hodgins. Reprinted by per...ission of Atheneum Publishers, an imprint of Macmillan Publishing Co. From *Limbo: A Memoir About Life in a Nursing Home by a Survivor*, by Carobeth Laird. © 1979 by Carobeth Laird. Reprinted by permission of Chandler & Sharp Publishing, Inc. From *Starting Over*, by Ernest Hirsch. © 1977 by Ernest Hirsch. Reprinted by permission of Christopher Publishing Co. From *Multiple Sclerosis: A Personal View*, by Cynthia Birrer. © 1979 by Cynthia Birrer. Courtesy of Charles C. Thomas, Publisher. From *The Magic Mountain*, by Thomas Mann, trans. H. T. Lowe-Porter, © 1927. Reprinted by permission of Alfred A. Knopf, Inc. From "Terminal Cancer and the Coda Syndrome: A Tandem View of Fatal Illness," by Lois Jaffee and Arthur Jaffee, in *New Meanings of Death*, ed. Herman Feifel. © 1977 by McGraw-Hill, Inc. Reprinted by permission of McGraw-Hill, Inc. From "Resolution: The Final Life Task," by Naomi Fiel, *Journal of Humanistic Psychology* 25, no. 2. © Spring 1985 by Sage Publications. Reprinted by pe˙ nission of Sage Publications, Inc. From "I Get So Lonely Out Here," by Maria Goodvage, *San Francisco Chronicle*. © 1988 by *San Francisco Chronicle*. Reprinted by permission. From *It's Always Something*, by Gilda Radner. © 1989 by Gilda Radner. Reprinted by permission of Simon & Schuster, Inc.

Credits Continued on Page 312.

Second paperback printing, 1997

Library of Congress Cataloging-in-Publication Data

Charmaz, Kathy, 1939–
    Good days, bad days : the self in chronic illness and time / Kathy Charmaz.
      p.   cm.
    Includes bibliographical references and index.
    ISBN 0-8135-1967-5
    1. Chronically ill—Psychology. 2. Self. 3. Chronically ill—United States—Interviews. I. Title.
    R726.5.C49 1991
    155.9' 16—dc20
                               90-28864
                                   CIP

British Cataloging-in-Publication information available.

Contents

Preface   vii

1   Introduction   1

Part I   Experiencing Chronic Illness   9

2   Chronic Illness as Interruption   11
3   Intrusive Illness   41
4   Immersion in Illness   73

Part II   Problems in Everyday Life   105

5   Disclosing Illness   107
6   Living with Chronic Illness   134

Part III   Illness, the Self, and Time   167

7   Time Perspectives and Time Structures   169
8   Timemarkers and Turning Points   196
9   The Self in Time   228
10   Lessons from the Experience of Illness   257

Epilogue   266
Methodological Appendix   271
Notes   279
Glossary   287
References   293
Index   307

Preface

Having a serious chronic illness often crystallizes vital lessons about living that otherwise may remain opaque. For many years, I have pondered over what people learn through experiencing chronic illness. I have long noted that having a lengthy, uncertain illness affects people's emerging self-concepts. I also have come to understand that studying the experience of illness illuminates elusive, evanescent meanings of time. A disabling, unpredictable chronic illness rips apart taken-for-granted daily routines. Many ill people find themselves relating to time in new ways. Some of them reflect deeply about their lives and about time. Their thoughts, feelings, and actions about themselves and about time clarify experiences that occur more generally throughout life. In this book, I look at how men and women make sense of having a serious chronic illness. I link their interpretations to their experiences of time and show how experiencing time provides latent lessons that foreshadow a new concept of self.

The genesis of this research is both autobiographical and intellectual. Ill family members, friends, and colleagues have all taught me about living with serious chronic illnesses. After graduating from college, I worked as an occupational therapist with patients who had physical disabilities. Despite the glowing words of rehabilitation rhetoric about maximizing human potential, I soon learned that my real task was to try to teach patients ways to manage at home that would keep them from the nursing home door. I also discovered that relearning the trivial tasks of self-care posed awesome hurdles, not simply in time and energy, but in reconstruction of the self. In those tasks, new, and often disquieting, meanings of self emerged.

Some years later, my interest in chronic illness and self resulted in a doctoral dissertation on those topics that focused on time and identity. Several of the ideas and a few of the interview quotations in this book come from that work. My dissertation research was also primarily based upon qualitative interviews, as is this current work. For the dissertation, I conducted 55 interviews with 35 chronically ill people. But I felt that those interviews just pointed the way for exploring issues about time and the self in chronic illness, rather than capturing them. In addition, the referrals for the study came almost exclusively from physicians who had close contact with those patients. After completing my dissertation, I wanted to pursue my interest in the experience of chronic illness, but I wished to gather more complete and richer data, and I wanted to include people with chronic illnesses who were less tied to professionals and medical care. Subsequently, I conducted 115 additional interviews of considerably more depth with 55 new respondents. Among them were several people who had not consulted physicians for years.

My research here differs from most interview studies because I talked with some participants over a number of years (5–11). It also differs in that I have had informal conversations with many of them as well as intensive interviews. Further, I have also interviewed twenty caregivers and providers and have amassed a collection of published and unpublished personal accounts and anecdotes about having a chronic illness. All these materials are reflected in the book, although I rely most heavily on the interview data that I have collected over the past eleven years.

The book focuses on self and time. Although earlier works on the experience of illness offer insights into both, they usually do so in the context of managing the illness, which is but one of my concerns here. My purposes include: 1) to look deeply into the experience of chronic illness, starting from the perspectives of ill people themselves, 2) to explore different ways that people experience chronic illness and to examine their implications for the emerging self, and 3) to show how the struggle for control over illness and for control over time is a struggle to control the defining images of self.

This work fits under the general rubric of social constructionism and interpretative social science; I examine how people with chronic illness create meanings of their illnesses and of themselves. My background in sociological social psychology and symbolic interactionism provides the theoretical underpinnings for this study. In medical sociology, the works of Fred Davis, Barney G. Glaser, Julius Roth, Anselm Strauss, and Irving K. Zola have most influenced me, and in social psychology, the ideas of Herbert Blumer, Norman K. Denzin, George Herbert Mead, and Ralph Turner have permeated my thinking. Anselm Strauss served as my dissertation chair; I gained much from his knowledge and wisdom.

To offer the reader some insight as to how people respond at different points in their illness and to different problems, I have assigned fictitious names to twenty-seven men and women and provided statements from them throughout the book. I have tried to record what people told me without revealing either their identities or those of other individuals whom they mention. With great reluctance and with much prodding of reviewers, I have shortened my interview excerpts and edited them slightly. Left to my own devices, they would have stood as is with every "ah," "um," and "you know" faithfully recorded.

In Part I of this book I present three ways that people experience illness: chronic illness as an interruption, intrusive illness, and immersion in illness. Each way of experiencing and defining illness has different implications for self and for meanings of time. Those meanings become stark when ill people must deal with the logistics of disclosing illness and living with it, which I cover in Part II. Meanings of time congeal for people with serious chronic illness and become attached to self more visibly than for other adults. In Part III, I examine meanings of time structures and the ebb and flow of time perspectives. I also include a description of timemarkers and turning points. Then, I specify the temporal conditions experienced during chronic illness that lead to anchoring the self in the past, present, or future. I conclude with a discussion of the lessons that we can learn from studying the experience of illness. These lessons focus on the effects of illness upon the self and the related policy implications of the research. A methodological appendix describes the research participants and outlines the research procedures. A short glossary of specialized medical and service delivery terms is included at the end of the book.

During my work on this study, I have presented numerous papers at professional meetings on these topics. I am grateful to the many colleagues who expressed interest in my work and encouraged me to complete it. The book was written in small increments and large jumps, when I could fit it around my work. I had written drafts of the first two sections of the book and part of the third section as of three years ago. As I revised the manuscript, I checked my ideas through further interviewing. I also came across works by Kathleen Lewis, Sefra Kobrin Pitzele, Cheri Register, and May Sarton, all of whom had chronic illnesses. Their experiences affirmed a number of ideas that I had already developed—sometimes startingly so, such as May Sarton's poignant longing to regain her lost self. I include occasional quotes from these authors to illustrate my points. But I developed the analytic framework for the book from materials gathered earlier.

Steve Charmaz, Adele Clarke, Dave Hoffman, and Katie Torgensen were particularly helpful in locating people to interview. Special thanks are due to the members of my writing group, Joyce Bird, Anna Hazan, Marilyn Little, and earlier, Adele Clarke, Gail Hornstein, Barbara Rosenblum, and Susan Leigh Star, for their interest in my work and for their critiques of chapters. Fran Bedingfeld, Steve Charmaz, Carol Engelbrecht, and Irving K. Zola also commented on individual chapters; Patrick Biernacki has been a valuable methodological consultant over the years. I have talked at length about these ideas with Carol Engelbrecht, Lyn H. Lofland, and Mona Partlo. Their engaging responses spurred my thinking. I am much indebted to Norman K. Denzin, Lyn H. Lofland, Gottfried Paasche, and Jane Prather, each of whom read the entire manuscript, discussed it with me, and offered helpful remarks on it.

For a faculty member with heavy teaching and program administration assignments, conducting extensive research is something of a luxury. Thus, receiving two grants from the Faculty Incentive Grant Program at Sonoma State University helped enormously and expedited this work. A sabbatical leave afforded me time to edit the manuscript. My writing has benefited from thoughtful comments and careful readings by David Bromige, William de Ritter, Helen Dunn, and, especially, Gerald Rosen of the English Department at Sonoma State University. It has been a privilege to work under their tutelage. I am grateful to the School of Arts and Humanities at Sonoma State University for inviting me to teach courses on writing, which prompted me to learn new ways of handling it. Mariana Chavez, Linda Cirk, Nancy DeLong, Linda Gaede, and Lillian Lee helped with clerical assistance at various stages of the work. I am fortunate to have worked with a professional editorial staff at Rutgers University Press, and I thank Marlie Wasserman and Kate Harrie for their efforts to produce the book.

Over the last ten years, I have discussed some of the ideas in this book with students in the Gerontology Program at Sonoma State University. They have always offered stimulating and supportive responses to my research; I thank them. My greatest debt is to the people whose stories appear in the following pages. I hope the reader senses their remarkable candor and the openness of heart and mind with which they talked about their lives.

In memory of Loraine Patnode Calkins

1

Introduction

I'm kind of up and down, but mostly better than I have been. This is like . . . a real strong summer for me. And, I have bad times. . . . If I overdo too much, but if I take it easy and I relax and I don't do anything like . . . lately it's just been like maybe a day and then I'm like a battery and I get plugged in and then I'm ready to go again. And a lot of my symptoms, they're kind of on and off and sporadic. . . . One thing that is really for certain—if I don't get my rest, I'm definitely feeling really, really crummy. And let's see, this year I . . . had two bouts with this that's lasted about a week to where . . . it was real difficult for me to even come down the stairs and [go] back up. But, with the sleep apnea and the medication on sleeping, and then I think of my illness. I think, "God, I could take this and I might not wake up in the morning." But then I think, "Well, if I don't take this, I'm not going to go to sleep." And if I don't go to sleep, I'm going to feel lousy, so . . .

Progressive gains. Plummeting losses. Plateaus. At forty-nine, Nancy Swenson experienced each phase during her eight years of debilitating symptoms from carcinoid tumors. When Nancy was very sick, her illness drained her of energy, pulled her into her physical self, obliterated her ability to concentrate, impaired her vision, and robbed her of sleep. Increasing her medications resulted in more symptoms, including lethargy and depression. From an overwhelming physical dependence to an independence that belied her condition, Nancy Swenson experienced the good days and bad days that marked her illness.

After two years of contesting negative decisions on her application for a disability benefit through Social Security, Nancy received a temporary benefit. She said:

1

> But then they evaluated me in a year. . . . They were almost going to take it away from me and then they talked to one of my—my counselor—actually . . . and she explained to them [that] I can't be something I'm not. I can't go in to [see] a doctor . . . without being presentable. . . . Then he's going to look at me and say, "God, she looks healthy enough, nothing wrong with her." And my counselor explained that I don't enjoy having this, and it's kind of demeaning for me that I'm not able to go out and participate and [be] in a full-time job and take care of myself. . . . So they sent me a letter saying that they will keep me on Social Security and SSI for three years, but then, at that time they will reevaluate me again to see where I'm at. So I just figure I'll take it a day at a time and cross that bridge when I come to it.

Living with a serious illness takes effort and devours time. It also means overcoming stigmatizing judgments, intrusive questions, and feelings of diminished worth. Nancy Swenson tried to plan her life to fit her illness. That meant balancing exertion with rest, simplifying daily tasks, and reordering time commitments. If she did not, she got sicker—sometimes much sicker. Nonetheless, others still expected her to function and to keep her household together. Nancy's serious episodes of illness caused havoc, because, like many women, she was the center of an extended family. She cared for her eighty-two-year-old mother who had Alzheimer's disease and helped several adult children who moved in periodically. Her unacknowledged illness shaped daily life for her mother, her children, her mother's attendants, and, sometimes, her tenants.

The structure of medical care extends its reach into the depths of private life.[1] Nancy had signed her property over to her children years ago, which made her eligible for Medi-Cal, the California Medicaid program. She had virtually no choice of physicians—she went to the only physician in her area who accepted Medi-Cal patients. Because she might need medical care—lots of it—in the future, she could not afford to lose her Medi-Cal status. Not for a man. Not for a marriage. Thus, the economics of medical care figure in relationship ethics. Nancy said, "I can't possibly ever get married because I'd lose Medi-Cal. No insurance company in this whole world would touch me unless I . . . went to work for a corporation. And then they probably wouldn't take preexisting illnesses. . . . I can't get married because I . . . could wipe somebody out. And I had a fellow I was seeing, and he . . . proposed and so I had to quit seeing him."

Not only does the structure of medical care shape personal decisions, but also the experience of illness leaves its imprint upon feelings, actions, and meanings of time. Having an illness and being a caregiver shaded Nancy Swenson's views of love, marriage, and her future. Because she had received so little acknowledgment of her illness, being with an attentive man gave her comfort. Yet knowing that her life was foreshortened had caused her to reevaluate how she used whatever time she had. Before she became ill, she had worked toward future goals. Afterwards, she sought valued moments and good days in the present. Further, she did not want to face years of caregiving again as her health declined. She commented:

> The last fellow was very doting . . . but he wanted to live my life for me. . . . He wanted me to rent my place out, to move in with him, get married, ah; he'd get a hot dog stand; I'd manage it. . . . And I'm thinking, "Wait a minute; that's not what I want at all." . . . And another thing, the man had a heart problem. And I thought to myself, "Gosh, what if, you know, he had a stroke? I could end up taking care of him like I'm taking care of my mother." And no way.

Though Nancy Swenson had little acknowledgment of her illness or help for it, some people demonstrated their concern for her. Her son paid several large bills that she could not handle. A disability rights counselor helped her appeal the negative decision for receiving a disability benefit. Two friends whisked her away occasionally for a care-free weekend.

Later, Nancy's mother became bedridden. With the help of attendants and equipment, her mother's care became far easier than when she was ambulatory. Meanwhile, Nancy's condition plateaued. She came to a sense of resolution about her illness and her life: "I do find now that this whole thing has brought— and with my mother—has brought so much peace into my life."

Life was not so peaceful earlier for Nancy Swenson, as will become evident in later chapters. She had to contend with having a disruptive mother, a chaotic household, a difficult foster daughter, troublesome tenants, and little money in addition to being exhausted, in pain, and, sometimes, incapacitated.

From getting through the day to dealing with the inequities of medical care, living with chronic illness can result in unending knotty problems and unforeseen hardships. Chronic illness can set people apart from others and take over their lives. Nonetheless, most people live with their illnesses rather than for them (Conrad 1987; Schneider and Conrad 1983). Often, they try to keep illness at the margins of their lives and outside the boundaries of their self-concepts.[2] Though sometimes people can do that, at other times they must struggle to do so, and at certain points they cannot.

In this book, I look at the crossroads between living with chronic illness and constructing a self. I study the private face of a public problem—what illness and disability mean to people who have them. Their meanings are imbedded in experiences of time. More than allowing time for illness, losing time to it, or reducing time commitments because of it, being ill gives rise to ways—often new ways—of experiencing time. Through interpreting elusive moments, critical minutes, lengthy hours, and slow stretches of time, people make sense of what their illnesses mean for their emerging selves. Hence, both meanings of illness and self take root in subjectively experienced durations of time.

Meanings of illness and self shift and change as illness progresses or recedes into the past. Further, the type, quality, and quantity of help that ill people have available to them affect how they experience time during their illness. Although some avenues for help might exist, many ill people neither know about them nor have access to them. Instead, they live with illness with little information, help, or even, psychological support.

Living with serious illness and disability can catapult people into a separate reality—with its own rules, rhythm, and tempo.[3] Time changes—drastically. A once calm day with a smooth schedule or a taken-for-granted routine now teeters with ups and downs. A "good" day permits an even schedule and is savored. A "bad" day forces attending to immediate needs and may be dreaded. Good days and bad days lend new meanings to the present and future and shade memories of the past.

Illness can become an odyssey to unfamiliar emotional and social terrains filled with passion, pain, and renewed purpose.[4] Ill people and their intimates enter worlds with concerns, feelings, and problems removed from conventional adult worlds. Yet for lengthy periods of time, many people live with a serious chronic illness and move between being immersed in it and keeping it contained. As they do so, their priorities change, and often along with them, their perspectives. These changes flow from experiencing illness and, simultaneously, inform it. What began as an alien reality, after months or years, may come to feel natural, unalterable—right. What may have once devastated someone can become a path to developing confidence, competence, and compassion.

Though living with chronic illness may mean entering and being swept away by a separate reality, more adults enter it as they age and as the incidence of chronic conditions increases. For that reason, we need to explore the experience of illness and to give voice to people who have it. My analysis stresses disruption, immersion, packed schedules, slowed moments, and problematic relationships, all issues in contemporary life. If so, then why study only people with chronic illnesses? Because the stakes for them are so high. Their gains are often small, but their losses are great. Studying the experience of chronic illness provides lessons about suffering and loss and about occasional wondrous moments.

Having a chronic illness means more than learning to live with it. It means struggling to maintain control over the defining images of self and over one's life. This struggle is grounded in concrete experiences of managing daily life, grappling with illness, and making sense of it.

The significance of the experiences of chronically ill people transcends chronic illness. Other adults who experience loss and crisis will find strong parallels with the experience of ill people. They, too, struggle with putting their lives together after disruption, controlling time, creating continuity with past selves, reconstructing new selves, devising timemarkers, noting turning points, and locating themselves in the past, present, or future. And so do people who have experienced divorce, acute grief, job loss, or who attempt to recover from addiction or abuse. Studying the experiences of chronically ill people provides a window for observing duress and change.

What does it mean to have a serious chronic illness? How does chronic illness affect the sense of self? What is time like during sudden crises, uncertain outcomes, long convalescences, and daily regimens? How do ill people make sense of timeouts for illness, slowed time for symptoms, added time for regimens, and crisis time? What mirrors of self does illness provide? And when do ill people take note of them? When do they resist accepting the images mirrored in illness? When do they accept them? How do feelings about illness become melded to periods of time, and moreover, to self? In which ways does illness provide timemarkers that locate the self in time? I address these questions in the following chapters.

In this book I look closely and deeply at the experience of having a chronic illness. I do not intend to trace the experience through particular men's and women's lives, but I do aim to give some sense of the general properties of that experience.[5] Certainly the results are tempered by the data I have collected, my interest in time and social psychology, and my awareness of what it takes to plan and to complete daily tasks that have become much harder and take much longer.

As a work in interpretative sociology, this book provides views from two different levels of interpretation: first, from men and women who reflect upon past experience or relate present experience, and second, from the sociologist who studies, synthesizes, frames, and creates an interpretation of these experiences. Moving between these levels results in choices and emphases (Denzin 1989; Geertz 1988; Marcus and Fisher 1986). I attempt to provide statements from people who have chronic illnesses to illuminate their lived experience on which the analysis rests.

To observe how chronic illness affects the self, we must look at the degree to which illness impinges upon ill people's everyday life—their work, homelife, free time, if they have it. In turn, how illness impinges upon them depends upon the structure of their lives and when and how they define illness. Moreover, both the degree that illness impinges and the social context surrounding it delimit the amount of control an individual can have. And that control is pivotal for the shaping of self.

Subsequently, in the following pages, I tell a story about experiencing chronic illness. Strands of the story are taken from fragments of ill people's thoughts, feelings, and actions, and then woven together with a sociological thread. The story reflects the social setting, times, and culture of the people whom I studied. Thus, themes of individual choice, responsibility—and blame— might resound more strongly here than in other parallel studies because these themes have resonated within the holistic health beliefs and practices to which a number of my respondents subscribe (cf. Crawford 1986; Lowenberg 1989).

Still, what I weave together here is a sociological story. Though I have tried to present ill people's experiences from their viewpoints, the rendering of them and the analytic framework in which I couch them remain my own.[6] In telling the story, I portray feelings as well as thoughts and actions, dilemmas and doubts in addition to hopes and happy endings.[7] To an extent, I have entered the worlds of chronically ill people and have compiled their stories to tell this sociological story.

P-A-R-T
I

Experiencing Chronic Illness

People experience serious chronic illness in three ways: as an interruption of their lives, as an intrusive illness, and as immersion in illness. The disease process usually remains elusive to them, and an illness trajectory (Strauss et al. 1984; Corbin and Strauss 1988) might seem abstract and removed. Rather, from their perspectives, illness disrupts their lives; it intrudes upon the day—frequently each day; it engulfs them.

Different relationships to time flow from each way of experiencing illness. A changed relationship to time and a changing body bring latent lessons about the developing self. Meanings about illness reflect the qualities of lived time, how much time illness takes, when it takes time, and what other time constraints press upon the person.

In Part I, I describe experiencing chronic illness as interruption, intrusion, and immersion. Some people experience illness in a straight-line progression, although that progression may take years. Their lives are disrupted—temporarily, they hope and often believe. Time goes on but symptoms remain. Symptoms, and, should they adopt them, regimens, cut into the day. Good days spawn hopes. Bad days dash them. More frequent bad days make valued pursuits difficult or impossible. Worlds narrow and health fades. Life becomes founded on illness when people cannot handle their former responsibilities. Their days change. Days dissolve into maintaining illness routines and weathering complications and crises—immersion in illness.

The movement from initial interruption to complete immersion usually occurs with both bumps and jolts and long smooth stretches. During those smooth stretches, illness remains in the background of people's lives. They may almost forget that they have a serious

9

chronic illness. But as the disease progresses, illness comes into the foreground again.

Not everyone experiences a linear progression of illness. Some people define intrusive symptoms long before they have a major disruption or crisis. Thus, their illnesses start in the background of their lives and move stealthily into the foreground as they demand more attention and time. Other people catapult from an initial interruption straight into immersion in illness routines. They suffer through a crisis and then find themselves at home sick—very sick. Similarly, a crisis may signal the beginning of a life founded on illness. If so, these people find that their health prohibits them from returning to their former positions and that they cannot create new niches for themselves. They slide into a life founded upon illness.

Certainly medical treatment can alter how someone experiences a chronic illness. Technical advances may permit keeping an intrusive illness in the background of life. Conversely, iatrogenic effects can bring it into the foreground.

Experiencing illness as interruption, intrusion, or immersion depends upon the person's definitions of the experience. Illness cannot exist without such definition, for its meaning derives from the person's bodily feelings, thoughts, and sentiments. In the subsequent chapters, I look at the experiences that influence ill people's definitions.

2

Chronic Illness as Interruption

I just cried and cried. And I think finally what got me out of this [feeling that she could not cope with having Hodgkin's lymphoma], one lady really helped me a lot . . . she had been sick in her life before. . . . She was so infected she almost died . . . and I thought, "If she can go through that at such a young age, I can do this [cope with the treatments] . . . that's mentally what went click, click, click in me.

I said [to myself], "I'm going to go through the steps [of radiation treatments for Hodgkin's lymphoma]; I'm going to drive myself to Garden General Hospital; I'm going to lay under the radiation beam for a minute and a half every day; I'm going to put my clothes on; I'm going to go home. I'm going to get done with this; I'm going to do it, finish it, get well, and get on with life." And from that minute on, that's what I did. Really I did. I just said, "That's it."

From shock to grief. Then resolve. Gloria Krause recounted her responses to her diagnosis. Devastated by the diagnosis and the subsequent surgery, she had resisted having radiation treatments. Hodgkin's lymphoma had taken over Gloria Krause's life. Everything had changed. Until she heard the other woman's story, she had languished in sorrow and wavered about going through the treatments. Afterwards, she defined her illness as temporary and resolved to recover.

Several other crises followed, each with major surgery. Then, the second episode of Hodgkin's:

I went through so much and then for this to happen again . . . [pauses]. But I truly believe that when this is all over and they get rid of this [the cancer], I don't think it will ever come back. . . . I think most of my friends and the people around me

11

don't look upon me as a sick person, because they know the situation is only temporary. And I think he [Greg, her on-again, off-again lover] knows that and that's what I told him; I said, "It's not going to be like this all the time, you know I am going to get well, and that's very important."

Disruption. Disbelief, then doubt. After Gloria's second surgery for Hodgkin's lymphoma, she faced radiation again—this time with massive amounts of chemotherapy. Nonetheless, she remained steadfast in her view that she had an acute illness to be battled and won. Then Greg confessed that he did not know if he could handle the possibility of cycles of illness and treatment culminating in death. Greg's fears undermined Gloria's views and dampened her hopes. When I asked her, "What did he say?" she said, "Well nothing really, he agreed and said, 'Yeah, that's true' [that the illness was temporary]. I just gotta go through the treatments, get it done and over with. I've got to get it behind me and past and go on and do what I want at that point. I want it to be over. I want to be able to look back and say, 'The treatments are finished.'"

Temporary crisis. Life-saving treatments. Full recovery. These words reflect how Gloria Krause defined her illness. Somehow she could not die, for, at thirty-four, her life had hardly begun. Chronic or terminal illness seemed too improbable—impossible.

Gloria took refuge in defining her illness as an interruption. By putting brackets around it, she felt that she had more control and could combat it. For a number of years, Gloria's experience replicated her definition of illness. Each time, crises, treatments, and complications temporarily engulfed her in illness. Then relative quiescence. Yet Gloria never fully regained her strength and vigor after her first ordeal.

Like Gloria Krause, many people start their journey through chronic illness with a crisis. Improvement and felt recovery may follow. Even if people with serious chronic illnesses do not begin with crises, they have crises later, perhaps much later.

Undoubtedly, having certain types of cancer such as Hodgkin's lymphoma can promote defining illness as an interruption of life. Having a condition such as congestive heart failure may not. Nonetheless, someone who has congestive heart failure might have similarly defined his or her heart disease for years.

What does defining illness as an interruption assume? In its clearest form, illness is temporary, of short duration, and with a predictable outcome: *recovery*. Hence, ill people expect to get better—soon. They have little or no concept of chronic illness and disability.

These beliefs assume a temporary present and an unaltered future. Complications? Unrelenting illness? Permanent disability? These outcomes seem unreal, or at least unlikely (Charmaz 1985a; McGrail 1978; Pill and Stott 1982). Should these nagging questions arise, ill people hope—and sometimes avow—that they will be spared such troubles. A firm vision of a positive outcome also results when ill people have won past "victories" over illness. They believe that they will recover again despite physicians' dire warnings. Hence, they view illness as something to struggle against and to defeat (Charmaz 1987).

How do definitions of illness as an interruption shape thoughts and actions? How do interruptions occur? What is time like? How does time during a crisis contrast with other experiences of time? Who witnesses the illness?

Looking for Recovery

Defining illness as an interruption means looking for recovery. Initially, it means looking for complete or nearly complete recovery; later on, it means looking to regain the last plateau. This definition is consistent with conceptions of acute illness and care, which commonly frame assumptions about illness, including those of many practitioners. Here, ill people adopt the status, expectations, and time perspectives of those who have acute, rather than chronic, illnesses. They may become living exemplars of Parson's (1953) "sick role," which is predicated upon assumptions of acute illness.[1] That is, they willingly relinquish ordinary adult responsibilities, become cooperative patients, and expect their physicians to cure them. For them, being ill equals being in the sick role.

Being hospitalized for a period buttresses this definition of illness. In fact, however, the hospitalization may signal a series of changes that identify people as chronically ill and propel them into the role of a chronic care patient. When seventy-nine-year-old Effie Kolb had a mild heart attack, she fell and soon found herself in the hospital with a broken knee. Her fall started a chain of events that led to her placement in a board and care facility. As she looked back, she said, "I never expected what [actually] happened; I never expected to lose my home. No, I just thought I was going to get well. I hated to break up my home, you know. I didn't think too much about that I wasn't going to get to live a regular life."

People like Effie Kolb do believe that recovery requires time. Taking a "timeout" to work on getting well or to wait for recovery grants illness a special kind of time, meriting a temporary halt of usual pursuits. Certainly devastating symptoms allow no other choice. In addition, physicians provide legitimate reasons or requirements for taking time out for illness. Patients make comments like the following:

> I have to take time to get back on my feet.
> I'll be good as new after I finish the treatments.
> My doctor says I have to take a leave so that I can concentrate on getting well.

With the timeout, priorities and pursuits shift radically. If everyone involved agrees that the illness is serious, the shift is complete. Consensus obligates ill people to take time out and to wait for recovery (Parsons 1953). Hence, they not only put their lives on hold, but also their identities.

A valid crisis may seem unrelated to *chronicity*. Typically, people define their severe onset as bona fide illness. But they may stop there. Real interruptions by illness include "when I passed out," "when I was rushed to the emergency room," or "when I had the heart attack." To them, being sick means being in crisis.

Assumptions about recovery and recovering self, i.e., retrieving a past self, presuppose imposing order on potential chaos and shutting out dark shadows—decline and death. More concretely, these assumptions also presuppose an active physician and a relatively passive patient. Further, these assumptions foster medical compliance. Thus, the patient may later feel betrayed when compliance does not pay off in recovery.

Beliefs in recovery as the sequel to illness take on moral imperatives. Ill people's "should" recover often shades into "merits" or "deserves" recovery. A number of people, including Gloria Krause, echoed this woman's comment: "I really feel strongly that once this [illness and treatment for it] is over, that's it, that I've paid my dues with my health."

Beliefs in meriting recovery follow earlier diagnostic shock (Clarke 1982) about having the illness at all. As a result, these ill people bargain with themselves and their practitioners (Charmaz 1980b; Kübler-Ross 1969). As Lorber (1975) says, they try to be "good" patients. They want to do the "right things" for themselves and by extension, their families; they do not wish to bear the stigma of illness or to burden their families (cf. Schneider and Conrad 1983). Being good patients buttresses ill people's beliefs that they have honored their part of the contract, however tacitly they bargained its terms. In their view, they have atoned for whatever prior failings or omissions for which they might have felt responsible. For them, being good patients means taking time out for illness. Having done so, they feel that they deserve to return to the activities on which their preferred identities and their "real" selves (Turner 1976) rest.[2] Hence, in their view, being ill means temporarily putting aside their identities and selves while they recoup and wait for recovery. Since they expect to recover, they feel no need to alter their conceptions of self for any length of time. In such cases, illness remains external to the self (Kidel 1988). Hence, these people view themselves as currently identified by temporary illness, but with their social identities awaiting them.

Certainly, having virtually no conception of chronicity can prompt people to look for recovery. A middle-aged woman had a diagnosis of multiple sclerosis for seven years and could trace episodes for eighteen years. She saw her illness as a series of acute episodes. She said, "It's like having a bad flu. Everyone gets the flu sometimes." This woman did have some continuous symptoms such as sporadic confusion, slight memory loss, loss of strength, and high fatigue. However, because she had no need for a rigid schedule and had always avoided intellectual tasks, her symptoms remained unobtrusive. Her definition of illness affected how she handled her condition. She said, "I should make a pattern of my vitamins and I should make a pattern of my exercise, and of my rest. But I guess I just don't think of myself as being sick."

Subsequently, this position can lead to acknowledging the presence of illness during an episode but to disassociating self-concept from it. Under these conditions, people feel as though they have been hurled into an unreal world. While there, they witness their bizarre symptoms and failing health. But they expect to return to their real world and real self. As one woman said, "It was almost like being in a dream world. You never really believe that you have something that's going to degenerate to where you couldn't walk. It was outside of me. I couldn't relate to it. I believed it—but didn't believe it [that it would last]."

The assumptions of acute care seem to work when ill people define only the *worst* episodes of illness as interruptions that merit professional attention. By adopting the model of acute care in this way, they resist having illness inundate their lives and their self-concepts.

All the foregoing views make sense, given the experiences of ill people. But often, practitioners believe that these views reflect their patients' denial of illness.

Constructing "Denial"

Why do some people act as if their illnesses are acute, when practitioners and the public see them as chronic? Why do other ill people discount medical information about their illnesses? Why do still others insist that their lives will go on exactly as before, even though they now have an impairment?

Denial of illness is the standard answer to these questions. However, an understanding of ill people's meanings of their illnesses and their actions leads to a range of interpretations of which denial is merely one possibility. Further, the concept of denial cuts off the very interactive and interpretative processes that lead to evaluations and judgments of it. Denial becomes something seen as inhering within the person rather than as a judgment pronounced about that individual or as a product of the interaction with him or her.

Denial is a label. Definitions of denial rest as much on judgments as on an ill person's behavior. Therefore, denial is an elastic category. It stretches (Charmaz 1980b). Judgments of denial decreed by powerful professionals stretch to fit their agenda, usually patient management and compliance. Professionals sometimes make hasty judgments of denial during fleeting encounters with bewildered, shocked, or fearful patients, who cannot communicate, or perhaps even articulate, their concerns at the time.

Responses indicating "denial" actually may reflect natural outcomes both of the structure of patient-practitioner relationships and of patients learning how illness affects their lives. When professionals believe certain patients deny their illnesses, they deny them partnership in treatment planning. And occasionally, they write these patients off early in the course of their illnesses (Charmaz 1987). By doing so, professionals may preclude these patients from receiving services or assistance later when they have learned what their illnesses mean.

Judgments of denial also pervade ordinary discourse about illness. Ill people, and their families and friends, increasingly adopt the language of denial. Hence, the attendant judgments of denial reach into intimate relationships and into self.

How do judgments of denial arise in illness? What it means to have a chronic illness is ambiguous in several ways. First, as implied above, many people hold sketchy and simplistic conceptions of their illness. Physicians themselves may feed their patients' uninformed views and sketchy conceptions. For example, Christine Danforth had seen a dermatologist for almost a year. She recalled:

Well, first he said, "[It was] photodermatitis," and he said that for a long time and then, he said, "No, discoid lupus." And I said, "What is it?" And he said, "Oh, it's just a rash." And he never really explained what it was. And a friend of mine told me a little bit because she had a medical background. . . . I said [to her doctor], "Somebody told me you couldn't sit out in the sun." He said, "Well, it's not a good idea." But he was real . . . it was like, "Don't question me."

Physicians may be forthright about the diagnosis but let their patients discover what the diagnosis might mean. Ron Rosato recounted, "I said, 'Well, what is this problem?' And they put me in a hospital and took a lot of tests, and they said, 'Everything is fine, Ron, but—so we've come up with multiple sclerosis, a possible multiple sclerosis.' I said, 'What is that?' And they said, 'You'll learn about it.' And I did."

If an initial crisis is all-consuming, it mitigates against thinking about progressive impairment or episodic cycles. During her first episode of multiple sclerosis, Heather Robbins had but one pressing question: "Am I going to die?"

The more esoteric the illness, the more likely the person initially lacks information and understanding about it. Like Ron Rosato, many of my respondents did not know what their diagnoses meant at first. A woman with multiple sclerosis suspected that she was having a mental breakdown because she did not know that double vision and forgetfulness were symptomatic of it. Another woman with lupus erythematosus expected to recover fully from her condition, if she followed her physician's orders.

It is hard to deny the "facts" of one's existence if one has neither the facts nor access to them. It is also hard to deny "facts" if physicians give patients contradictory information or if different physicians' recommendations cancel each other out. Sara Shaw abandoned medical supervision entirely for five years. She said, "After I realized the doctors didn't know what they were doing, I did much better [on her own regimen]. *The doctors don't know.*"

Furthermore, people who had esoteric illnesses seldom could get facts from fellow patients, mainly because they did not know anyone else with the same condition. Nancy Swenson said, "Only one in 2,000,000 get this disease, so I've never had the opportunity to meet anyone else who has it." Family or physicians sometimes prohibit independent information-seeking, particularly at the onset. Several people with neurological conditions reported that their physicians expressly told them not to read anything about their conditions because of inaccuracies. When a middle-aged woman received a diagnosis of multiple sclerosis, she asked her physician about joining a self-help group. She said, "He told me, 'I don't want you to meet anyone. Only the worst cases go to those meetings.' "

New treatments and surgical procedures sometimes reverse or extend the course of previously "hopeless" conditions. Some patients then say, "I'm cured," but do not realize that from a medical perspective they still need to follow a medical regimen. Like others, a middle-aged man said, "My heart condition—I don't have a heart condition any longer—the surgery cured that." Certainly physicians' enthusiasm for particular procedures or treatments occasionally convinces patients that their distress is temporary (Petch 1983; Radley and Green 1987).

Medical breakthroughs raise hopes that a miraculous intervention might emerge if one can hold on long enough. Several people said, "There's always hope of a cure." Such hopes stress dramatic improvement or recovery derived from equally dramatic means. Further, hopes for the future undermine motivation for taking present action, which is predicated on a continuing illness.

Definitions of illness may foster responses that look like denial. What stands as a bona fide "chronic" illness? Criteria for chronicity sometimes become murky in specific instances. For example, the course of cancer can vary from an acute or chronic to a terminal illness. And five-year "survival" rates become reinterpreted as "cure" rates, which, in turn, promote definitions of episodes as acute. With such ambiguity, no wonder that ill people choose the most optimistic definition.

Further, the course of a chronic illness may be atypical. Stories abound of patients whose "miraculous" improvement defied all their practitioners' predictions. Such stories feed hopes—and hopes spawn judgments of denial. Yet I found several people whose personal dramas matched myths of miracles.

In addition, long periods may elapse during which an illness progresses slowly. For example, a woman of fifty-seven had been diagnosed with multiple sclerosis thirty-five years earlier.

Prior to experiencing a major exacerbation, she had treated episodes of her illness as interruptions without much serious or lasting consequence. Hence, for most of her adult life, she defined her illness according to her experience of it.

Definition and experience of chronic illness dialectically affect each other. A view of oneself as only having a minor ailment or occasional bouts of serious illness can last if the illness is episodic. At those points, illness comes to the foreground, but otherwise it remains in the background. Four years after going on heart medications for frightening symptoms, Vera Mueller said, "I don't think about it at all; it is very much in the background now."

Definitions of illness may merge with beliefs about the power of personal motivation. In turn, these beliefs may be judged as evidence of denial. A number of people believed that thinking positive thoughts about recovery, keeping a positive attitude toward self, not giving in to being sick, and the like would shape the outcome of their illness. Lara Cobert's progressive symptoms resulted in a diagnosis of myasthenia gravis. She said, "I kind of believe that as soon as you accept something, that helps make it so. So I was not about to do that. I didn't want to close any doors. I never—George [her boyfriend] used to point out [that] I'd say, 'The doctors said I have myasthenia gravis.' I didn't say, 'I have myasthenia gravis.' "

To the extent that people do not experience their altered bodies in their own worlds or to the extent that they can define impairment as temporary, they will not view their conditions as chronic. Their stance looks like denial, but it derives from the reality of their experience. Because part of the issue of denial derives from how and when others make such judgments, professionals should broach legitimate questions of denial only after an ill person has had time to experience his or her body in its altered form.

Certainly, the possibility of denying illness still exists. If ill people persist in defining their illness as acute, but it long continues, they plant the seeds for denying illness. Likely, these people stretch their "allowable" duration of an acute illness, because they do not wish to acknowledge that illness has become something more than an interruption.

Learning about Chronicity

Weeks and months of unrelenting symptoms teach ill people about chronicity. Further, learning about chronicity means discovering its effects upon daily life. By attempting to manage their usual activities, ill people discovered the meaning of their altered bodies. After his first heart attack, Harry Bauer recalled that "when I was laying on the bed there [at the hospital], I told the doctor I was going to go back to work. He said, 'No way.' He said, 'When you get up from there, you'll find out how weak you are.' I used to be able to pick up 100 pounds in each hand. When I got up from there, I found what he meant, I couldn't hardly hold myself up."

The meaning of disability, dysfunction, or impairment becomes real in daily life. Until put to test in daily routines, someone cannot know what having an altered body is like. Heather Robbins did not have her first serious episode until ten months after her diagnosis. But others mistook having a diagnosis with dealing with the disease. She recounted:

> People said, "You deal with this so well [immediately after diagnosis]." I just said, "I haven't really dealt with this because I haven't been ill." I mean you can't deal with something until you've experienced something, uh, you don't have to. So as soon as I got sick with it and had to deal with it then, that I think is when I realized I had MS [multiple sclerosis]. . . . Now I am learning where I can go and how much I can do without knocking myself out.

The yardsticks of the past, not of an altered present and future, measure distances to walk, tasks to complete, and plans to make. Lessons about chronicity come with discoveries that those yardsticks pose arduous or impossible standards.

Frequently, ill people must abandon their hopes and plans, and relinquish their former activities. Illness and disability force lowering expectations of self—at least for awhile. Yet doing so shocks and unsettles people. In his book, psychiatrist Clay Dahlberg recounts his feelings when he learns that he can go home after having a CVA [cerebral-vascular accident]: "That was a glorious day. I started planning all the things I could do with the incredible amount of free time I was going to have. Chores I had put off, museums and galleries to visit, friends I had wanted to meet for lunch—so many joyful things. It was not until several days later that I realized I simply couldn't do them. I didn't have the mental or physical strength and I sank into a depression" (1977:30).

The difference between past and present functioning contrasts sharply, for the past remains so close. After a few days of convalescing at home, Dahlberg tried to work on several of his usual projects. He states, "I wanted to do some necessary house repairs and work on my amateur sculpture, but shortly discovered that I had neither the physical nor mental ability to do much. Sculpture requires concentration over a period of several hours and I was just not up to it. A repair also, even a small one, demands a steady hand and I didn't have it" (1977:41).

When ill people return to work, the "before and after" contrasts become striking. These contrasts call into question their sense of self and undermine their taken-for-granted notions about their capabilities. For example, a middle-aged woman with heart disease had been known as a fast worker in her unit. When she returned to work, after having had a serious heart attack, she discovered that she could not complete her work on time, let alone early.

Even if ill people's work has been modified, they may learn that they need more help. However, the social repercussions of requesting help may prove too costly. Here, learning about chronicity includes learning about stigma. Lin Bell, a middle-aged woman with heart disease, worked as a janitor with a team of men. After her first bypass surgery she said:

I have a lifting restriction on me at work and if the guys see— they're always coming by and saying, "Now you take it easy" and we have these great big barrels that we roll around and fill with trash and stuff and if they see me going, heading out . . . to the dumpster to dump that, they're right there, real protective. But I won't ask. I don't want any special treatment. I don't like to be treated as less than I feel that I am.

Rather than face chronicity, some people will go home or even retreat to bed and wait until they recover. They expect to awake one day and once more reclaim their past selves. Here again, assumptions of recovery make illness simply a way station between prior and future states of health.

Yet for others, the meaning of illness as interruption is less stable. As they experience their bodies in time and space, they learn that this episode means more than a brief interruption of their lives. With this realization, they redefine their illnesses and what they need to do about them.

Defining Interruptions

Defining any interruption means that ill people, or their families, think about the illness. They treat it as a separate event, distinct from other events. Usually, they seek help. People come to define illness as interruptions in four ways: 1) experiencing disruption without diagnosis (multiple sclerosis, lupus erythematosus, 2) suffering a rapid escalation after vague symptoms followed by crisis (heart disease, epilepsy), 3) being stricken with a sudden severe onset (myocardial infarction, CVA), and 4) getting bad news from unexpected test results (cancer).

Disruption without a diagnosis is jarring. For a time, ill people may account for a disquieting incident or strange sensation by viewing themselves as under "stress" or as suffering psychological duress. To the extent that physicians spark or concur with their reasoning, they seldom seek further explanation until their conditions worsen.

Because she accepted her doctor's view that she nearly had a "nervous breakdown," Cynthia Birrer only remembered the following episode long after she received a diagnosis of multiple sclerosis. In addition to the vision loss she describes below, her symptoms included a staggering gait, quivering hand, numb foot, and complete exhaustion. She writes:

It all began, I think in 1967. That was when I first became multiple sclerotic. Now I well remember that day in late October. . . .

Feeling quite sick, I walked listlessly into the gray shed that housed the overnight book loans. Whatever it was did not pass. Reluctantly I took my place in the scheduled room. Picking up the question paper, I gave a moment's thought to the time-honored injunction to read it carefully. Dismayed, I found that I could not read it at all. I held a single sheet of paper whereon two blurred, indistinctly typed images overlapped . . . separated. I cursed. How could I allow an exam to upset me like this? I covered my left eye but that was no good; the faint letters slithered hither and thither. (1979:60)

Accepting a doctor's diagnosis ends the search for explanation. Recurrent symptoms, however, can result in people believing themselves to be ill though their doctors can find no physical cause. Several people even had physicians who agreed that they were too ill to work. Yet these ill individuals could not apply for disability assistance because they did not fit the accepted categories.

Lacking the physician's validation of illness is even more troubling. People with esoteric illnesses often felt that their physicians portrayed them as feigning illness, either by magnifying insignificant symptoms or by psychologically inducing physical distress. The feeling of being discounted and distrusted intensifies when family and friends share the physician's view. Doubt multiplies. When everyone else doubts that ill people are sick, they even begin to distrust their own bodily sensations.

Diagnostic relief follows a late diagnosis. When a physician finally identifies the problem, these ill people often first respond with relief and gratitude for receiving a seemingly dreadful diagnosis. A middle-aged woman with a metabolic disease said, "Thank God. At last I *know* it is something real."

The diagnosis gives these people legitimacy, restores others' faith in them, and, moreover, renews their belief in themselves as having genuine feelings and valid complaints. At last, their conditions can consume the attention that others had riveted on their fragile selves. At last, they might receive the help they seek. They prefer facing a devastating diagnosis to defining themselves as neurotics, malingerers, or shirkers.

Whether these people previously blamed their psyches, physical beings, or physicians for their distress, they had suffered from profound discord within themselves and within their worlds. When that discord lasts for months or years, the lack of validation shatters their trust in themselves and their perceptions. Not only may these men and women accept their diagnoses, they may embrace them. Having a diagnosis gives respite to a shaken self.

Commonly, amorphous symptoms eventually worsen or another more alarming symptom develops; illness rapidly escalates (Locker 1983). An older woman had had Reynaud's phenomena for years, but only after she developed a severe rash did she begin to suspect that she had lupus erythematosus. A young woman had had spells of extreme dizziness. She discovered that her balance and coordination were so poor that she could not ski. Then she became frightened and sought help. After her physician diagnosed her as having multiple sclerosis, she looked back through the past and found several other episodes that could have been multiple sclerosis. Like Cynthia Birrer's (1979) experience with it, she could now reinterpret the past in light of the present diagnosis.

If troublesome symptoms, even pronounced ones, do not last, people often do not seek help. Lin Bell first had frightening symptoms five years before her heart attack. But they soon subsided and her other symptoms remained vague. She recalled:

> We went up to Tahoe on vacation and all of a sudden I felt like a cement truck was falling over me. . . . And then I got real scared and so we got in the car to come back home, because I didn't want to go to the hospital up there, I wanted to die in Santa Maria. Half way down the mountain, I felt terrific, so I lit up a cigarette, you know, and then we had a fight because—so I wasn't going to go to the doctor 'cause I felt fine once I got off that mountain. And finally I went to the doctor, oh, about four days later. And that's when he started me on Inderal and all that blood pressure [medication].

A rapid escalation reduces self-blame, if professionals had discounted vague symptoms. Lin Bell's physician had diagnosed a mild angina. But her symptoms mysteriously worsened:

I passed every treadmill test I ever took. You know, I last—I do great on them. But then . . . I just got terrible angina pains one night. . . . So I went in the following Friday. . . . He [her cardiologist] had asked me if I could be bringing this on myself and I said [that] I didn't think so. Because it happened, you know, when I went to bed—I mean why would you want to bring something like that on you when you're going to bed for a good night's sleep? I said, "I don't—I don't think so, Dr. Martin." And it made me feel like he thought I might be a hypochondriac. . . . My mother . . . enjoys poor health, so I was just crushed thinking that I was becoming more and more like Mother. . . . So when he took me in for the angiogram and they were looking, you know, up at the screen and stuff, he says, "Oh Lin, you're— you're not imagining anything. One of your arteries is almost 90 percent closed." And I said, "Oh, thank God!" I was so happy because I knew I wasn't like Mother.

Lin Bell had had disturbing symptoms long before her doctors discovered anything definitive. An older man with heart disease only had a "funny feeling on my face, which didn't happen again" before his heart attack. His doctor tested him for a blockage and found nothing, but told him he had had a ministroke. Ten days later he had severe chest pains. He said:

I hadn't exercised for about four months so I went to the gym and I did aerobics, real hard . . . came home and an hour later I was in the hospital. So that brought it on. . . . It was a tightness and, I couldn't breathe and on the way down there, I started perspiring. . . . I said, "Dave [his son], take me to the hospital," and he says, "Do I have time to take a shower?" And I said, "No." Anyway, it was very funny. . . . And then on the way down there, I thought he was going to crash into somebody and I said . . . "We want to get there," you know. So he races the car up to the door, and they open the door and bring a guerney out and David's still behind the wheel and the nurse says, "Don't let him drive into the lobby." They thought he was going to drive right in in his little car! Anyway, it was, ah—I almost died laughing.

Despite preceding symptoms, someone may not view his or her rapid escalation or crisis as marking a chronic illness. Even sophisticated patients sometimes permit medical terms to obscure the meaning of their conditions. Medical historian Ilza Veith made sense of earlier mysterious bodily sensations when she diagnosed herself as having had a cerebral-vascular accident. Her physician confirmed her self-diagnosis. She writes:

> No one in the world can imagine how grateful I was to hear the expression "cerebral vascular accident." It seemed such an elegantly youthful affliction as compared to "stroke," which I had used all along in my private conversation with myself. A stroke denoted a drab condition of elderly, if not to say, old, patients, and there wasn't anything scientific about it. But CVA had that learned elegance and—innocent as I was at that time—suggested a matter of impermanence. (1988:18)

Rapid escalation. Quiescence. Improvement. Cycles that include some improvement foster optimism despite more severe episodes. Further, someone may not believe that a present setback points to permanent disability and thus resists adopting any symbols of it (cf. Duval 1984). An elderly woman's unsteady gait resulted in a prescription for a cane. Rather than buy one, she decided to rent a cane. "That way I'll work to keep it [her illness] temporary; I'll *have* to give the cane back."

Frequently, ill people limit their activity and autonomy rather than tacitly affirm that they have suffered further physical losses. To them, acknowledging decline symbolizes an intolerable assault on their self-concepts. Illness threatens to leave a permanent stigma.

A sudden onset of illness can cast people in the patient role immediately. They lose consciousness, have seizures, or lose control of functions. However, even a sudden onset is a *process* rather than an *event*. If people can view their symptoms as trivial, albeit unpleasant or painful, they usually do so. Consistent with Cowie (1976), men with initial heart attacks sometimes normalized them for several hours or more before seeking care. For example, a dentist recounted:

> We had two of my grandchildren and my son and his wife for dinner and it was a very stressful day. . . . So, when they left, I had a little bit of what I thought was indigestion. And ah, I went

to bed and I couldn't sleep and I had this pain and I took some antacids and got up and sat up and listened to the television . . . and finally, the pain got more severe in my stomach. . . . And I—I suddenly found that I couldn't close my teeth together. Being a dentist, I know that one of the signs of coronary attack is disarrangement, apparently, in the jaw so you can't put your teeth together. So I thought, "Well, it's happened."

Getting bad news, such as an unexpected serious diagnosis, can catapult anyone into crisis. An ordinary adult becomes transformed into an ill patient. Frequently, these crises come without warning through test results. A medically constructed interruption develops in three ways: 1) previous normalization of symptoms (Davis 1963; Wiener 1975), 2) gradual discovery through testing, and 3) unsuspected validation of illness or crisis.

Niel Fiore describes getting bad news: "It became apparent that the lump was not going away by itself and should be examined by a doctor. . . . I had come in for antibiotics for what I had hoped was simply an infection but, without ever checking with me, he was talking about removing my testicle for precautionary reasons" (1984:2–4).

A few people I interviewed had had vague symptoms but normalized them. They did not seek medical advice for them, per se. Rather, their physician found evidence of illness during a routine physical. For example, a young woman had a physical before entering nursing school. Afterwards, her physician told her that she had severe diabetes, which necessitated a complete medical workup in the hospital. Previously, she had blamed her anxiety, fatigue, and weight loss on working too long, studying too hard, and dating too often. This woman felt surprised and embarrassed that she had not correctly recognized her symptoms.

Shock diminishes with multiple tests despite lack of physical distress. But physicians may offer reassurance that further testing means nothing. One woman's doctor requested that she have another X-ray in a month, just to check the first X-ray. She did not suspect anything, although as a former medical technician, she knew more than most patients. Sequential tests, signs of illness, and interactional cues raise suspicions. This woman began to suspect cancer when her husband told her to call her doctor after having the second X-ray. She felt rising panic, "I just had that sense of being in two places; I mean it was like a high tight place I was in."

Further positive test results increase the person's suspicions. This woman recalled having the X-ray: "Because I came in from out of town, the doctor processed it . . . right away and they told me something was there. I cried; there was all sorts of things that it might be; it might not be cancer. So I had to go in and have a [test] that same day. There is something called calcification which it might have been. . . . But it wasn't."

Such episodes may seem entirely removed from ill people's selves and their bodies. They feel shock and disbelief one moment and loss and grief the next. Their anxiety mounts as each test confirms their worst suspicions. As one woman remarked, "as far as time seemed concerned, everything seemed interminable. Every wait, every wait for every report from every test was intolerable."

The Experience of Time

What contributes to different experiences and perceptions of time during initial and continued disruptions of illness? When do ill people attend to time? Clearly, the type of onset, ill people's preconceptions about illness, their lives, and their actual illnesses all affect how they experience time.

Elusive Time

How ill people experience time depends, in part, in how they experience their symptoms. When ill people gradually accommodate to vague symptoms, the present seems almost the same as the past. Moreover, if others' help automatically increases, then both illness and a changing experience of time remain muted.

A recently retired husband, for example, gradually relieved his arthritic wife of tiring housework. Although her illness had progressed, she still experienced it as sometimes interrupting her life, but not as intruding upon it. Because of his help, she marked time in large chunks and did not need to gauge her activities against clock-time. Here, experiencing occasional interruptions, having her husband's help, and having a slow progression of illness coincided to forestall changes in her experience of time. In contrast, such changes occur rapidly when symptoms disrupt life and no one offers to help.

When a crisis follows slow progression, ill people may explain a formerly elusive relationship to time. "No wonder doing everything took so long." "Now that I look back, I realize that I was cutting back on my usual activities." "I had slowed down."

Waiting Time

Defining chronic illness as temporary fosters experiencing time as waiting time. Yet ill people's situations shape their experience of waiting and their emotions shade it. Thus, different types of waiting emerge. Sometimes people experience each type of waiting sequentially, perhaps in rapid succession.

To begin, an assured outcome means waiting for an affadavit certifying health or promising recovery. If people do not define themselves as presently or potentially ill, they simply carry on as usual while waiting. They preserve an earlier tempo and time perspective with little sense of emotional disruption. When they first receive medical attention, these people wait for concurrence of expected good news. For example, a woman's physician ordered a biopsy for a lump in her breast. Because she had none of the predisposing factors, she assumed that the lump was benign. For her, the waiting meant validating her assured outcome.

Here, waiting derives from bureaucratic rituals removed from ordinary life. Waiting becomes annoying dead time. Thumbing through boring magazines in the doctor's office fills empty time. Lying under a paper cover alone in a chilly examining room for half an hour wastes time. Standing in long lines at a clinic is frustrating and grating. The meaning of waiting lies in the irritating concrete experience of it. Waiting time means lost time and a loss of control over time (cf. Schwartz 1975).

Although these people believe that they will have an assured outcome, they do wait. To them, seeking medical care and following medical advice attest to taking responsibility for their health. Only in this limited way does waiting touch their self-concepts. They place their real selves in the immediate past. For them, waiting is only incidental, soon to be dismissed and forgotten.

In contrast, acknowledgment of possible or present illness causes perspectives and experiences of time to change. The period of waiting means the time necessary to pinpoint problems or to create recovery, whether by "fighting" illness and "taking" responsibility, or by becoming a patient. As people increase their fight against illness, time quickens. As passive patients slow down to the sick role, time also slows down.

Like an assured outcome, an improbable present distances self and feeling from unfolding events. Yet events do unfold and from "objective" views portend of bad news. "What? Can this be happening to me?" The events ill people experience seem surreal—unreal. Recent events have thrown them into another reality without warning. Like Dorothy in *The Wizard of Oz*, they feel catapulted into an alien world in which events remain dissociated from them. They wait to get through the present so that "real life" can go on in the future just around the corner. Since the present seems so improbable, they wait for it to end and with it, the shadows of illness. Until then, they wait.

An improbable present occurs when a person waits for reassurance that symptoms or earlier tests mean nothing. Joanne Dhakzak recalled being diagnosed with Hodgkin's disease: "I was in such a daze. I didn't believe that it was happening to me—because when I went to the doctor, I said, 'I don't know why I'm here. There's nothing wrong with me.' Maybe that's why it came as such a shock when the doctor said I had Hodgkin's."

Is it cancer? Could it be angina? Pangs of uncertainty spring up when current, frequently undiagnosed, symptoms could mean a serious chronic illness. Avowals that current symptoms are temporary and mean nothing are pierced by nagging doubts, silent questions, and fleeting moments of dread and fear. Much fear and anxiety may hide beneath a social face. Long moments of doubt and fear lead to focusing on self. When people disallow their fear, they may dive into their usual routines. Waiting ranges from disquieting moments to a distressing ordeal.

Pangs of uncertainty develop as one discovers bodily changes, cues from other people, and facts about the disease. As clues accrue, what may have began as passive, rather complacent, waiting ends in uncertainty and dread. As uncertainty grows, fears sometimes become worse than later realities. Someone may fear a brain tumor but the condition turns out to be multiple sclerosis (Robinson 1988b). Someone else may fear heart disease but it proves to be ulcers.

When pangs of uncertainty lead to fear and dread, people wait to know, to be sure. They wait for information. They wait for change. They wait for telling symptoms to develop. And they wait for them to subside. Between signs and clues, time stretches into a long, empty duration. Time stops. These people become locked into a protracted limbo. The self swings between an anchored past and an uncertain future. A woman said, "I felt . . . that—'I don't have anything; it's silly. It's nothing. What am I getting all upset for? Why be a hypochondriac and what if I do and I probably do [have cancer] and then what will I do?' And my life is just falling apart. These two fears go on simultaneously or alternately back and forth a great deal." A recurrence of past diagnosed symptoms fuels suspicion quickly. Inch by inch, pangs of uncertainty grow into dread and fear.

In contrast, an agonized waiting means excruciating psychological and/or physical suffering *now*. Waiting means getting that time over and regaining control of self and life. Illness and treatment overtake these people. Time slows. Waiting seems endless. Another woman faced the uncertainty of a recurrence of cancer. She said, "It was dreadful; those were the longest days. I couldn't concentrate on anything else."

Unlike most people, Gloria Krause made no distinctions between an agonized waiting and conventional clock-time. For her, rather than time stopping, her world stopped. When describing her round of chemotherapy, she remarked:

> It [time] was like anytime—it was the same. It's just like right now. It's like everyday life. It's—time is just time. It didn't seem long; it didn't seem short. Of course, I just wanted to get it over with. And I'd call my doctors and I'd say, you know, "When?, what's going on?, what's happening?, when's this going to stop?" And they'd say, "You've just got to ride it out." So it was just a matter of waiting. . . . When I was sick, I—you know—the world stopped. It was a real helpless feeling, though, a real helpless feeling.

Whatever their views of time, people ache to end this waiting and long to put it into the past, or to forget it.

A dreaded future may coincide with agonized waiting. The future, as well as the present, remain unsettled and undetermined. The dreaded future engulfs the present self. Likely, someone puts his or her self on hold. The self experienced now—be it a grumpy, fearful, martyred, apathetic, or withdrawn self—becomes a temporary self. The past self remains insulated and protected. By being held in abeyance, the past self remains less contaminated and muddied by illness. Then, should the news be good, the person can resume being his or her past self. Thinking about resuming the past self gives solace in the ambiguous present and reduces the sting of the dreaded future. Doing so may also provide a time buffer during which a person can begin to adapt to change.

Crisis Time

Crises are founded on disruption, immediacy, and immersion. In crisis, a radically changed present separates from the past. Like a guillotine, the crisis severs the present from the past and shatters the future. Hence, ill people feel severed and swept away from their pasts into an uncontrollable present and future.

The actual interval of time between the immediate past and

the present crisis is brief. However, the immediacy and immersion given in crisis lengthen it. Quite clearly, a subjectively experienced crisis also necessitates remaining alert and involved in what happens. This awareness and involvement yank people out of the past and force them into the reality of the present (cf. Flaherty 1987). Otherwise, crisis may be externally imposed but subjectively experienced as an improbable present.

Gloria Krause believed that her previous episode of Hodgkin's disease precipitated her bleeding ulcer. Her story illustrates a rapid shift from past to present, and how more serious crises successively topple upon each other. Gloria's crisis occurred while she was already in intensive care. However, she dreaded shifting from medical treatment to surgical intervention. To her, it meant changing from a qualitatively different past to a dreaded present. She had hemorrhaged four times in five days. Each time staff thought that they had stopped her bleeding. Then, she hemorrhaged again. Facing yet another surgery threw her into a new and more horrendous crisis than the past five days of intensive care. For her, facing surgery again seemed worse than facing death. She recounted:

> I cried and cried and said, "Dr. Overby, I don't want surgery because it takes you so long to heal from surgery." . . . and they did a scope and he—I mean his eyes looked at mine and he said, "Gloria, the hole in your stomach is as big as my fingertip." I mean I had a *hole* and the blood was going out of this body . . . and I was just begging him not to have surgery. . . . He said, "The bleeding is not going to stop. You have to have surgery— you have to go in." . . . I mean he looked at me with such seriousness in his eyes, you know, and I knew, and I said, "When are we going?" It's like you're not going to think about it, the decision has been made. And you are not going to rebleed and rebleed and rebleed. He said, "You're going into surgery right now, right now." I mean it was like midnight.

An agreed upon crisis immerses everyone involved in the present. Durations speed up when involvement increases in amount and intensity. When people feel overwhelmed by the enormity of crisis, they handle it in small pieces by concentrating on the details.

During a crisis, the present teeters with uncertainty and the future seems remote. While drawing participants into the exigencies of the present, a crisis simultaneously pulls people into a future. But they cannot reflect about what this future might reveal. Thus, images of the future remain vague and elusive. Moreover, when fear of death clouds the future, other, perhaps more accurate, images of the future may be precluded.

A crisis allows people to delve into the present and to *avoid* thinking about what looms in the future. Carobeth Laird, an elderly woman with multiple medical problems, writes, "As long as I was in a precarious condition, I didn't think of the future" (1979:14).

Although a crisis engulfs everyone in the present, paradoxically, it can offer them relief, a reprieve, from the immediate past. Immediately after suffering a CVA, Eric Hodgins recalls, "Once in the hospital bed I had a sense, almost, of elation. Here I was, and everything was somebody else's problem now. Whatever I had to do within the next immediate days would not get done and it wouldn't be my fault. Some problems that had been troubling me deeply for months would now not get solved; I was out of commission and my helplessness was almost pleasant" (1964:13).

For years, Gloria Krause had struggled to make a living by selling used clothes while she tried to develop a modeling career. She also struggled to form lasting ties with Greg, who flitted between her and another woman. When another crisis removed her from her struggles, she observed, "There was no pressure on me at all; that was kind of nice." Becoming eligible for a small disability benefit eased her earlier worries about how to pay for food and rent. One whole set of nagging pressures evaporated.

A crisis or sudden onset is a searing disruption. Loss. Profound loss. The disruption not only attests to loss of health, it threatens loss of self and way of life. The loss may force dreaded changes of relationships. Thus, a searing disruption casts unwelcome shadows on the future—long shadows.

Audiences of Interruptions

Other people watch what happens as someone becomes ill; they become audiences. They also play important roles. They affect whether illness becomes defined at all, whether it is defined as an interruption, what type of interruption, and what, if anything, it means. As observed earlier, ill people grant some individuals much more credence than others in defining the onset of illness. Credibility turns on authoritative status, type of relationship, amount of concern, and possession of information. Other people certainly affect *when* an individual defines possible illness. An elderly woman ignored her symptoms until her daughter insisted that she seek medical attention. Men commonly sought help only after their wives nagged, cajoled, or even threatened them. One wife whose husband delayed and refused said, "Oh yes, he went to the doctor after I told him, 'If you don't go, I'm leaving.' "

Defining illness is pivotal for those whose lives are interwoven with the person. Wives, particularly, scrutinized their husbands' behavior for signs of sickness. Subsequently, their persistence in defining illness resulted in their husbands' medical workups, hospitalizations, and consultations with specialists. A gay man's diagnostic search eventually led to chronic fatigue syndrome. He said, "Two of my friends were sure I had AIDS. They were really important in getting help. I was so out of it then [he had experienced confusion and disorientation]."

Once illness is defined, family and friends play crucial roles in monitoring it. When they learn how to define symptoms, they may prevent or forestall potential disruptions from occuring. For example, one woman's astute observations saved her husband from another stroke. The disruptions can be social as well as physical. A middle-aged man discovered that his uncontrolled anger toward his young children routinely occurred when his blood pressure skyrocketed. Taking his medication caused his blood pressure to drop and his temper to fade. Having that information eased conflict in his family and, simultaneously, prompted his wife to monitor his condition.

Ill people weigh their audiences' reactions against their symptoms, immediate concerns, and responsibilities. All are played out against the backdrop of their prior conceptions of illness. Hence, an ill person may be pushed and pulled in different ways. For example, Lara Cobert's friend and her elderly father both pushed her to seek help. But her own prior conceptions of health and illness and "natural" inclinations fostered delay. Another trusted friend, a nurse, bolstered her decision not to seek help. Lara said, "Well, see my friend's a nurse, and she's a really good nurse, but when it's her own friend she tends to— she doesn't want to scare you. . . . And she said it was probably just short-term and to watch it so I mean, you know, I really trusted Pam [the nurse]. So I just watched it for awhile."

Lara Cobert's primary audience, the nurse, justified handling disturbing symptoms like Lara had handled past acute illnesses. For her, illness provided a handy excuse when she had too much to do. Otherwise, she did not allow herself to be sick. Her harried life combined with her ideas about illness disinclined her to define it as interrupting her life. Lara remarked, "I was raising four kids by myself and working at this and that, anything, you know. I was too busy to notice too much."

Throughout the entire course of illness, ill people distinguish between private and public audiences. Private audiences generally know the latest news of someone's illness and how he or she thinks, feels, and acts about it. Public audiences only know slices of this person's experience. They may know the diagnosis but little or nothing about what the person thinks, feels, and does about it. Sometimes, however, a public audience has scant knowledge about the illness but witnesses how the person deals with it. For example, a neighbor of an elderly man only knew that he had diabetes, but unlike his daughter, knew that he drank heavily because she saw his bottles in the recycle container.

By its very nature, illness remains a private, family affair for many people. Their relative willingness or reluctance to provide friends and associates with details measures the degree of intimacy that they feel. However, they may reveal more to their practitioners than to acquaintances or associates. Hence, some public audiences become private. Events can throw nurses into telling moments with patients. Physicians occasionally know more than spouses and adult children about how illness interrupts a patient's life. A hairdresser may know more about an elderly woman's health than her adult daughter.

Absent audiences form shadow figures who ill people believe could materialize and dominate their lives. For example, a divorced woman had another serious episode but tried to define it as a minor disruption. She did not want to give her ex-husband cause to reappear and take the children.

Other audiences do not play their expected roles. Rather, they remain uncommitted, uninterested, or after several crises, expended. Occasionally, people have an illness or face a medical procedure that they believe disrupts their lives. But their friends and family do not. For example, the daughters of a heart patient discounted his latest crisis for his fear had resulted in more panic, rather than heart, attacks. Continuous emergencies (Robboy and Goldstein 1987), whether "real" or feigned, psychological or physical, self-induced or physiologically determined, grind away most sources of help and recast them as distant audiences.

Public audiences remain concerned and involved as long as they also can define the illness as a single interruption. But if it continues or reoccurs, their interest wanes and their attention dwindles. Furthermore, an initially sympathetic audience may even become antagonistic as their stance shifts from sympathy to irritation to condemnation. A middle-aged man gleaned that his co-workers thought he received undue favoritism from their supervisor. Although initially concerned, steady customers later terminated their orders from a salesman who was recouping from a heart attack. A nurse's co-workers assisted her when she first came back to work, but when she did not regain her earlier speed, they requested that she be transferred off the ward. In short, victim-blaming occurs when illness challenges the audience's taken-for-granted notions of temporary inconvenience and recovery.

As the ill person expands informal networks and seeks more help, professional involvement escalates. In a young woman's case, greater and more serious entanglement in medical and welfare institutions resulted. She told of seeking welfare assistance:

I thought they would give me the money to live on since it was obvious I wasn't able to work so they suggested a colostomy which was *horrendous* and they also, when I turned that down, said that they would send out a woman to talk to me. . . . I didn't have any formal thing done but she would come once a week at lunch time and talk to me at work and I *hated* that—I wasn't getting any money . . . and so the next thing I thought to do was to go back to the hospital and say, "Look I still have it," and they said, "Fine, we have to run you through the tests again because there's a chance you've gotten an ulcer by this time."

Occasionally, quasi-public audiences not only know about the person's illness, but also may allow the person to be sick. Private audiences may not. Joanne Dhakzak, who had Hodgkin's disease, lived separately from her husband in order to receive treatment at the major medical center several hundred miles from their home. She said that he could not accept her infirmity from surgery and radiation. Nor could he understand why her trailer was untidy, the dishes unwashed, and the laundry unsorted. So on weekends when he visited, she was "well." She hiked, attended movies, and explored restaurants with him.

Her actions resulted in three consequences. First, the staff knew and understood her reduced physical state and decreased stamina better than he did. Second, his attitude spurred her to feel responsible for herself and her recovery.[3] Third, she risked her health, even her life, to meet his expectations. For example, she hiked with him in deserted foothills while she still had stitches from major surgery. By her own account, had those stitches ruptured from exertion, she surely would have hemorrhaged to death.

Private audiences vary over time as the structure, relative intimacy, and geographical distance of the ill person's relationships vary. For example, Goldie Johnson's adult children had moved away years ago. When she became sick, her third husband planned her care. Her younger daughter, a home health aide, discovered that Goldie was overmedicated and that her husband planned to put her in a nursing home. She insisted upon moving Goldie to her own community. The daughter said, "I figured I cared more about her than he did. I would have done something sooner, but being two hundred miles away, I didn't know what was going on." Goldie's husband was soon stripped of any decisionmaking power since she divorced him upon relocating.

Thus, a shift in private audiences can result in radical redefinition of illness and of ideas for handling it. Goldie Johnson's story illustrates how an incurable condition can be redefined as an immediate crisis meriting amelioration. Shifts in private audiences, particularly when aligned with physicians, can construct or deny, expedite or delay, stress or obscure definitions of illness. As a result, what the ill individual experiences depends upon whether powerful external definitions coincide with his or her bodily sensations. And in sum, to the extent that powerful others deny, delay, or obscure definitions of illness, the likelihood increases that ill people will also discount their symptoms and themselves or, at most, define their sickness as a temporary interruption.

3

Intrusive Illness

What's a good day now? There is no good day. . . . Well, a good day now is sort of a neutral day. That's you know, there are never days when I have . . . almost never when I have lots of energy and run around! . . . I really don't pay that much attention [to my body], and never have. I do pay more attention now because I am limited [by severe emphysema]. . . . I don't know if you could say I monitor; I observe [laughs]. Yeah, I'm forced to observe it.

It's [his emphysema] accelerated . . . I mean there has been a decline in the last couple of years from Point A to Point B but I haven't noticed all that much. . . . I'm doing less than I did before . . . right before I moved here. But, you know, living within the parameters [here] you know, you just don't notice it. But on reflection, I think that it probably has been. . . . I don't have the vitality that I did. . . . Up until I was in my early forties, I kept my world view and my view of myself as a young person. . . . And now, it's, you know, pretty radically different as far as I am concerned . . . all of a sudden [I] see myself as an invalid [laughing], you know, an old invalid.

I asked, "How is that for you?" He said:

It's no picnic [laughing]. Yeah, I guess you come more to grips with your mortality and it's not that I'm afraid of imminent death or even long-term—I don't think about it that much, but . . . it makes me realize that there is not an endless life ahead of me. . . . My God, here I am in this position and . . . it'll be a lot tougher to get out of than formerly. . . . I don't know how much more time, you know, I could have a bad winter and get pneumonia and die. . . . I have a hard enough time breathing without that so . . . I see my dying as much more of a possibility than I did a few years ago.

41

Slow in pace. Low in energy. Short of breath. John Garston's former daily round receded into the past as his emphysema progressed. His apparent ease in moving around his tiny cabin belied how hard he found it to walk around his favorite flea market, or to climb a staircase, or even to manage the short distance to his mailbox. At forty-six, John's aging rapidly accelerated and death drew closer.

John Garston's illness had become intrusive. He could not ignore it. It cut into his life and circumscribed his choices. Nonetheless, he tried to live with it (cf. Fagerhaugh 1975).

What is it like to live with unremitting symptoms? What are "good" days and "bad" days? How do people accommodate and adapt to their intrusive illnesses? What stances do they take toward having an intrusive illness? How does being ill affect relationships? How do ill people try to keep their illnesses contained?

An intrusive illness means that the effects of illness continue; they do not simply disrupt ill people's lives temporarily. Granted, definitions of intrusiveness differ. What one man or woman defines as intrusive, another might define as a routine inconvenience, to be wholly discounted, and still another might see as causing immersion in illness. I take felt and defined intrusive illness as my starting point.[1]

From ill people's views, an intrusive illness forces them to accommodate to it, or to suffer the consequences, which can be both immediate and devastating. How they accommodate to their illnesses shapes whether or not they can live as they choose.

Definition of Intrusive Illness

An intrusive illness demands continued attention, allotted time, and forced accommodation (see Charmaz 1984; Corbin and Strauss 1988; Locker 1983; Maines 1984; Schneider and Conrad 1983; Strauss et al. 1984). When intrusive, illness becomes a permanent, if not always salient, part of life. People learn to expect symptoms and treatments, and to plan around them.

These people struggle, often successfully, to minimize the intrusion of illness upon their lives.

Though specific symptoms and episodes may be unpredictable, illness has become predictable. It affects people's daily round of activities (Brooks and Matson 1987; Locker 1983; Morgan 1988; Peyrot, McMurray, and Hedges 1987; Plough 1986; Reif 1975; Schneider and Conrad 1983; Strauss et al. 1984). Keeping an illness a secret becomes troublesome, even when it is invisible. In addition, intrusive illness takes time—for symptoms, for symptom control and prevention of flare-ups, for handling prior activities more slowly. Consequently, illness forces a new awareness of and relationship to time (Maines 1983).

Simultaneously, illness forces self-consciousness. Symptoms or episodes jolt active individuals' awareness of illness. They know, feel, and account for their intrusive illness. A young woman with multiple sclerosis described her intrusive symptoms in this way: "if it's like when I am really tired or something, I just simply can't do as much. . . . My leg won't work or something, and I just fall a lot."

Thirty-six-year-old Christine Danforth still worked despite having lupus erythematosus, Sjögren's syndrome, and the residuals of a serious back injury. In addition, she had to attend night classes to remain qualified for her job. Here is her account of how her conditions affected her:

> There's a lot of things I can't do. . . . When I go to night school . . . I have to go straight home to lay down before I do, or I can't go, where, you know years ago I wouldn't have had to do that.
>
> And I have really had problems with lights. I can't be in a room that has fluorescent lighting without wearing special glasses. So, if I go to class at night and I have to sit there with sunglasses on, then that makes me even more tired. It makes my eyes swell shut. . . . And I've also missed three classes and before I've never missed class.

Intrusive illness threatens control over self and situation, and results in uncertainty (Bury 1982; Locker 1983; Robinson

1988b; Skevington 1986; Strauss et al. 1984; Wiener 1975). When people define their illness as intrusive, they often view their control over it and over their lives as tentative and limited. A threat of loss of control also threatens loss of self (Charmaz 1983b). Thus, these people work to manage their illness and thereby exert more control over their lives.

Setting markers of acceptable levels of illness leads to defining anything further as overly intrusive. For example, a young physician with diabetes informed me, "The only time I get pushed out of shape is when I have to get up (at night) and give myself a shot. I get annoyed, I see it as an intrusion; otherwise, I don't. Then I have to figure out what to do."

Experiencing Intrusive Symptoms

Experiencing intrusive symptoms disrupts usual activities. Discomfort or potential threat of illness remains constant and cannot be dismissed (Bury 1988; Cobb and Hamera 1986). Two years before Vera Mueller began taking heart medications, she had intensified cardiac symptoms precisely when demands upon her escalated. She said, "I just don't want to think about it [her heart condition] and I resent it now that it keeps intruding into my way. It gets in my way."[2] I asked, "How does it get in your way?" She replied, "I have to think about the chest pains. *They are there.* I have to think about the fact that I haven't slept in two days. I have to think about the fact that, whoops, I didn't eat anything and I am smoking too many cigarettes and that I shouldn't be eating all this salt and that maybe I'd better make an appointment with the doctor and getting me to the doctor is like pulling teeth."

Intrusive symptoms permeate routine activities and interrupt the rhythm of the day. In short, symptoms cause problems that spread, like a cold in a grammar school class. Heather Robbins disclosed, "I have a problem; if I do trip, I can't catch myself. I know I'm going to land on him [baby] one of these days, or [on] her [toddler]. I've already stepped on her numerous times and things like that. . . . I feel terrible [about it]."

Experiencing intrusive illness leads to efforts to control symptoms and to prevent further symptoms and problems from developing. In turn, symptom control often requires constant effort. Frequently, social, rather than health, reasons spur this effort:

So I can continue to parent.
Because I don't want to be out of work again.
To keep my ex-husband [an abusive alcoholic] from getting the kids.
So I *never* have to ask for help [public assistance] again.

Controlling illness means controlling time and, moreover, emerging identity. By controlling identity, people maximize self-worth. That means keeping illness in the background, rather than in the foreground, of their lives. One way to control intrusive symptoms is to rest. Many of my respondents had to work (cf. Brooks and Matson 1987). They structured their day to enable them to keep their jobs, using any free time to recoup from work. Christine Danforth remarked, "I always try—like if I have to do something or I have to go somewhere, I try to do it always on Saturday. I like to leave Sunday to stay home and do nothing, because if I do something on a Sunday, even if I have Saturday free . . . it really makes me tired the rest of the week."

Resolving to preserve independence and self-worth encourages many people to try to control symptoms and, occasionally, the disease, and to avoid acute illnesses.[3] At times, the strategies themselves spur a chain of events that end in immersion in illness. For example, a woman took more medication than prescribed to mask her symptoms, although doing so accelerated her disability, which caused her to become housebound within two years. If someone's fragile control over illness shatters, then all the ways of trying to have a valued self flounder. Acute conditions drain strength and endurance, and therefore control over intrusive illness plummets. Not only does health deteriorate further, but also, the ill self, which had managed illness more or less effectively, is lost.

"Accepting" Intrusive Illness

What does intrusive illness mean to ill people? To what degree do they accept it? What does acceptance mean? Is it, as commonly believed, a necessary prerequisite for moving on with one's life? Both having the illness and attempting to continue a former life raise questions about "acceptance." In turn, the degree of acceptance suggests crucial assumptions about intrusive illness. Acceptance means agreeing to one's status without struggling and without envy, sorrow, or anger (Kübler-Ross 1969). I discovered four ways people respond to illness in relation to acceptance.[4] They ignore illness, they struggle against it, they reconcile themselves to it, and they accept it. Ignoring illness means overlooking it, or more accurately, looking over and beyond illness. Few people who try to continue a packed life can ignore direct discomfort or subsequent symptom management, though they may not handle either in medically approved ways. However, people rather readily ignore an invisible condition with vague, or minimal, symptoms, at least for a time (Siegler and Osmond 1979). Several men with emphysema and heart disease echoed this man's statement, "Mostly, I ignore it until it gets in my way."

Suffering or infirmity forces noticing illness when it interferes with or limits valued activities. John Garston said, "So I ignore it when I don't feel bad, you know, which is not often. . . . I mean if I'm just sitting here, sometimes I'll be wheezing; sometimes I won't. But if I get up to do anything, I'll naturally feel it. So I do ignore it quite a bit less than I did before."

Other people struggle against their illness (Charmaz 1987). A cerebral-vascular accident left a sixty-year-old man with a right-sided paralysis, slurred speech, and aphasia. But it did not dampen his hopes for and his efforts toward a full recovery. Though occasionally he could not control his anger about his condition, he vowed that he would struggle until death, if need be, to regain his speech and mobility. His CVA became his personal enemy to confront, to challenge, and to conquer.

When Bonnie Presley discussed acceptance, she had had lupus erythematosus for two years: "I'd rather be making a lot of money and I'd like to have more energy, but I've reached a balance and I've accepted an illness and I'm working around it. When I'm tired I—I go to bed. Even if it's at 2:00 in the afternoon." I asked, "What does acceptance mean to you?" She replied, "Accepting that I'm not what I used to be." One year later, her health had improved and she had revised her stance on acceptance: "I have to admit that I accepted it and after I got over accepting it, I think it was then that I started thinking, 'Do I really have to accept this? Isn't there anything I can do?' "

As Bonnie Presley's remarks suggest, acceptance shifts and changes as experiences, plans, and prospects change. Certainly the extent of illness, type of treatment, and current prognosis affect acceptance. So does the type and amount of support someone has. For example, a middle-aged woman reported that her lover dreaded her possible heart surgery because the scars would repulse him. As a result, she too rejected the procedure.

People may avow that they accept illness when it remains quiescent. Ill people may also accept some residual disability, as they learn to live with it, but they are unlikely to accept sudden declines with uncertain improvement. Patricia Kennedy remarked:

Don't think that I've been real passive about accepting this [her multiple sclerosis] because I haven't and I don't think I've gotten to accept it . . . and I don't know, Kathy, if I ever will. I accept it really fine when I'm in remission, [imitates her offhand stance then], "Oh, I have it" [and it's nothing] but not when I'm . . . not when it interferes with my life, when I want to go to class, when I want to study, when I want to do something other than be in this space [home].

Most people reconcile themselves to their illnesses. Reconciling means tolerating illness. It means acknowledging and handling pain, slowness, or fatigue. It means following a regimen or creating a routine to manage or mask the symptoms. In short, people decide to live with their illness (Corbin and Strauss 1988). They acknowledge the presence of their illness and attempt to accommodate to it. John Garston stated: "I just found it easier when I stopped fighting it." Another man remarked, "I can live with these symptoms, if that's all."

Hence, acknowledgment of illness lies within "acceptable" limits or boundaries. Accepting anything beyond those boundaries seems beyond human capacity. These views spawn tacit bargains to devote time and effort to handling illness within the set limits. People who do so often had bargained earlier to keep the first interruption of illness limited to one episode. At this point, they resign themselves to the presence of illness and bargain about the *extent* of it.

Lara Cobert refused to accept a foreshortened life and progressive disability from myasthenia gravis. Five years after her only episode, she said, "Usually, people die of complications. . . . But I never thought about that [dying] very much because I never really accepted it. Suddenly, there's an immediacy about putting effort into getting well. . . . The future becomes dealing with the disease."

When ill people reconcile themselves to their illness, they may do so only as they experience it in the immediate present, but not the future. Thus, a man declared: "I can tolerate this situation for a short amount of time, say two years, but at the end of it, that's it." In addition, ill people may reconcile themselves to one set of symptoms or routines but not to others.

Reconciling oneself to illness differs from accepting it. Reconciling means accommodation to the extent that these men and women can tolerate. "I adapt to my illness now. In that way, I adjust to it, but I'll never accept it." Acceptance shapes the future as well as the present. It assumes accepting the identities others deem to be "appropriate" for them (Charmaz 1987). In contrast, reconciling self to illness means rejecting identifying stereotypes others cast upon those with chronic illness. These ill people also reject practitioners' pronouncements that strip them of hope. "You will get worse." "You'll end up in a wheelchair." "There is *no* cure." Though she had reconciled herself to multiple sclerosis, Patricia Kennedy said, "I look for a cure."

Examining the degree of acceptance reveals ill people's views of self and their implicit theories of identity (Charmaz 1983b; Strauss 1969). Their degree of acceptance reflects the amount of assault upon the self that they can tolerate. Further, it reflects their limits of defining self and of being identified by others.

"Good" Days and "Bad" Days

Dividing life into "good" days and "bad" days provides one measure of experiencing an intrusive illness and a part of the taken-for-granted lexicon through which illness becomes understandable and explainable. Differentiating good and bad days in illness reflects a more intensified, focused version of evaluating days more generally such as in work, child care, and love. Good days and bad days also implicitly concede the limits of self and reveal images of self. Telling identifications emerge. What assumptions lie embedded in good days and bad days? What kind of experience do the terms denote? How does a "good" day, contrast with a "bad" one?

Most fundamentally, ill people define good and bad days according to their evaluations of the amount of intrusiveness of illness. The relative presence or absence of symptoms figures here. Ill people weigh their symptoms as they learn which ones they can dismiss or ignore. Certain symptoms may remain more or less present but vary in severity and intrusiveness. Hence, the amount of suffering and infirmity that ill people experience differentiates good and bad days.

Subsequently, suffering and infirmity create other important criteria for evaluating the day, such as the amount of time taken for illness and regimen. In addition, the kinds of activities possible, amount of productivity, degree of choice, and amount of control all figure heavily in evaluating the day. These criteria flow from the initial assessment of the amount of intrusiveness. When intrusiveness is low, most people have more choices and can exert greater control over them and over themselves. Conversely, when intrusiveness is high, choices narrow, and ill people have less control over them and over themselves.

Intrusive illness may lead to loss of control (Schneider and Conrad 1983). The relative visibility, embarrassment, or stigma produced by illness or the subsequent loss of control can significantly define a day. Feelings of control, and therefore of personal competence, shape whatever definition one makes.

Definitions of good and bad days result from juxtaposing and comparing one day with another. Decided disjunctures between the types of days lead to developing precise, explicit definitions of good and bad days. An elderly woman with cancer remarked, "Today's a good day, but yesterday was hell."

Evaluations of days are fundamentally intertwined with evaluations of self. Ill people measure the quality of the day against the self they recognize, acknowledge, and wish to be. Thus, they judge whether the day is consistent with the self they wish to affirm and to present to others.

A "Good" Day

A good day means minimal intrusiveness of illness, maximal control over mind, body, and actions, and greater choice of activities. Ill people concentrate minimally, if at all, on symptoms and regimen during a good day, or they handle them smoothly and efficiently. Illness remains in the background of their lives. Spatial and temporal horizons expand and may even become expansive during a good day. When illness abates, people have much better days. Like ex-convicts just released from jail, they may wish to make up all at once for lost time.

A single mother's temporal horizons had consisted of physically getting through the day and financially keeping her children fed throughout the month. Her spatial horizons had been limited to the distance between her bed, the bathroom, kitchen, and living room in her tiny apartment. When she began to have good days, her temporal horizons lengthened to ideas about how she wanted her family to live in the next few years and what kind of a future she desired for herself. She exclaimed in wonder, "Before, I dragged through the day, wondering if I could get through it. Now I have a whole life in front of me." During her past bad days, she had felt locked into an uncontrollable present. As the possibility of a long future stretched out before her, she began to see a chance of exerting control over it. In short, expanding time horizons characterize a good day.

Good days are, of course, relative to an ill person's criteria and experience of chronic illness. For some people, a good day means functioning as they had before illness became intrusive. Quiescent or controlled symptoms contribute to feeling relatively "normal" between exacerbations. Definitions of a good day shift and change according to the progression of the illness. For Patricia Kennedy, who had had debilitating flare-ups of multiple sclerosis, "A good day means to be able to get up and get out of bed by myself, to eat breakfast, to shower, now it means to go off to school, to participate in class, to rest and then go on [with household and family tasks]."

Definitions of a good day derive from a sense of being in character, being the self one recognizes and acknowledges. On a good day, ill people have more opportunity to be the selves they wish to be. In addition, on a good day, the earlier jarring questions about present self, the doubts, the eroded confidence, and the nagging fears about the future all recede into the past, or may be completely forgotten.

A "Bad" Day

A bad day means intensified intrusiveness of illness, less control over mind, body, and actions, and limited choices about activities. Illness and regimen take center stage. On a bad day, people cannot ignore or easily minimize illness. Further, their intensified symptoms may then elicit uncontrolled feelings. Christine Danforth, the receptionist with lupus erythematosus and Sjögren's syndrome, described a bad day: "I find that I'm really a lot more tired than, you know, if I just have a regular day. I have a lot more memory loss, ah, frustration and then I get depressed and angry. . . . I just blew [up] that day."

Frustration marks a bad day and leads to fury, often at self. Lara Cobert recalled her bad days:

My speech would slur a little bit, I get really pissed off, or I'd go to pick something up [and drop it] . . . I mean I got *really annoyed* when I dropped things and that was counterproductive only it didn't do me any good to get annoyed. George [her partner] would point out that getting angry at myself didn't do anybody much good. It's hard to accept things like that and you don't want to accept them on one level or on the other, there's no point at being angry. So, I guess I felt angry at myself, at my body.

Spatial and temporal horizons shrink on a bad day. When people take for granted that their activities will be curtailed, they voluntarily limit their spatial and temporal boundaries. When they struggle to remain active, they test and measure exactly what their spatial and temporal boundaries are. Patricia Kennedy stated, "On a bad day I can't get up, I have to stay home—I have no choice. I have symptoms—yes, [no] strength, lack of balance. It's hard for me to go out—I only go to safe places. Thrifty's [a store] too crowded—too many visual stimuli, too confusing. Somebody may knock me over. . . . On a bad day either I need to go with someone or take a cane. I know I should stay home and rest. On a real bad day, I can't do anything."

Like many other ill people, Patricia Kennedy graded bad days. Her definition of bad days changed when her illness flared. She commented, "I deal with time differently and time has a different *meaning* to me." She added that, "being sick is a waste of time," because it profoundly reduced time for tasks or for personal goals. Bad days elicit anger and frustration because they negate being one's preferred self. Bad days reflect a frustrating and frightening self, a self that limits the present and might foretell the future.

How do people handle bad days? They revise expectations of self and of the day downward. For example, some ill people try to use the day for undemanding tasks. By revising the day downward, they try to prevent bad days from becoming "lost" days.

Spatial and temporal boundaries can shrink so radically during a bad day that ill people seem to sink into self. In turn, their boundaries for interacting and functioning steadily contract. As people sink into self, they experience a kind of self-involvement that probably feels alien or distasteful. Under these conditions, people feel *out of self.* That is, the self presently experienced bears little resemblance to someone's "real" or "ideal" self. Hence, ill people often say, "I'm not myself today."

By saying to her housemates, "I am not myself today," a young woman with colitis alerted them to her bad day. She and her housemates had tacitly agreed that she needed to make no other verbal acknowledgment of her illness than such a statement. Through informing them, she requested them to reduce their expectations of her. Their acceptance of her illness and the ways she handled it minimized possible strain.

Not everyone, however, is able or knows how to smooth strained interaction (Davis 1961). Instead, fear, anger, or self-pity consume these people. Their immediate self-concern floods other interests and ordinary interaction. They feel that they cannot attend to conventions and courtesies. Family and friends may not understand the ill person's experience, or may discredit it. "He gives into it; he's being a baby." "Everyone's disgusted with her, she won't do anything for herself." Subsequently, these people have to contend with all the negative responses to them and whatever feelings those responses evoke in self precisely when they are having a bad bout of illness.

Shifting Criteria

Criteria for good and bad days shift as someone's condition improves or worsens. Good days become much better as health improves or treatment works. Earlier, ill people may have "normalized" discomfort, fatigue, or pain that permeated even their good days (Davis 1963; Wiener 1975). Thus, how much better they feel startles them. Six years ago, Vera Mueller had some bad days. Receiving medication and losing weight revised her days upward. She said, "Health-wise I'm fine. Actually I gained thirty pounds and then dropped fifty. I feel good, better than I have in years; I feel strong. . . . I'm more active; I don't get tired. The weight was really weighing down on me and I was having a lot of chest pain I didn't acknowledge. I didn't know it was there. I didn't realize it was there until it was gone. [Relates her wonder.] 'Oh it doesn't hurt. Oh, how surprising.' . . . I've just got a *ton* of energy I've never had before."

As illness progresses, this process works in reverse. A bad day gets worse—sometimes dramatically so. Similarly, the criteria for a good day also shift downward. Ironically, an earlier bad day can become a good day. For an elderly man with emphysema, a bad day eight years ago was a day when he experienced shortness of breath and fatigue when out in the yard. Five years later, a good day meant being able to move from the bed to his chair. Similarly, John Garston observed, "What used to be bad days [laughing] are—now, they are good days . . . but the quality of things, I think, is declining, you know, from, say a couple of years ago when I didn't think about it that much. And there would be isolated days when I had a lot of congestion and things like that. But that's all."

Cycles of quiescence and flare-ups foster noting how meanings of a bad day change. Patricia Kennedy explained:

> My daily regimentation is altered during exacerbation in that it takes me longer to do everything. It takes me longer to get out of bed, I have to get out, sit on the side of the bed, then get up. It takes me longer to shower. It takes me longer . . . because I just move much slower. And then as the day progresses, I have to build into that day [that] which I do all the time, an exercise program which takes . . . say an hour currently . . . it takes me an hour and a half to an hour and forty-five minutes; it's a big chunk of the day. Often, during exacerbation, I need to lie down and allow myself to rest for two hours a day and at that time, also, I need more sleep, I need twelve hours of sleep a night. My day is shortened . . . by what I need to fit into the day. Then, in addition, it's shortened because activities take me longer. . . . My time is almost regulated by the symptoms of exacerbation.

Patricia Kennedy had to take her symptoms into account; they intruded upon every part of her day. Whether or not self and others acknowledge bad days is crucial. Lesser bad days allow for more elastic definitions. What an ill person will allow to stand as a bad day, what significant others will confirm, and what everyone defines as a bad day can vary. For example, a woman did not discern a bad day until her symptoms became quite marked. Neither she nor her husband could tolerate sickness or sick people, so she neither talked about it, nor even defined it, until she was caught by it. (She also could plan and pace her day almost exactly as she wished.) Thus, the social context and meanings of illness shape definitions of good and bad days.

The social structuring of the day can turn a good day into a bad one. For example, Christine Danforth might have started a day feeling all right. However, the structure of her day expended her physical limits and mental acuity. The day moved too fast for her. Too many distractions disrupted her concentration and impaired her productivity. She began to have memory problems and made mistakes. She could not handle the flow of work. She remarked, "It's [the work day] sometimes worse on days where most of our staff now are part-time, which makes it a lot harder on me because when they're not there, I have to take more messages and more lengthy messages, so I get very frustrated and I have bad days when that happens."

When a cloak of silence surrounds illness, participants will not talk about the bad days until they are in the past, even when their actions acknowledge them. If someone's health takes a turn for the better, then others' acknowledgment of the earlier bad days becomes apparent in their congratulatory remarks founded on astute comparisons of the person then and now.

As illness grows more intrusive, bad days become certain, expected, and predictable. Yet exactly when they will occur and where they will lead remain unpredictable. These properties give an interesting twist to the concept of uncertainty. Ordinarily, it refers to progression of illness from the vantage points of both the physician's prognosis (and often, treatment choice) and the patient's experience of debilitating symptoms. But in these cases, "uncertainty" is persistent, continual, and anticipated—"certain".

May Morganson, who had renal failure, described her unpredictable, yet certain, bad days in these words: "Fortunately, it doesn't happen too often. I mean, you know, it's not like *every* day, every day after dialysis. But it's sometimes one or two days a week. And then lots of times they'll—in fact quite often, the dialysis patients have to have blood transfusions. And usually, I don't feel very well for a couple of days after a transfusion."

Though May Morganson could not predict exactly which days would be bad days, she did develop a timeframe for them.

Later, she disclosed that in fact the bad days occurred each week, and lasted for several days. As a consequence, she remained sick much of the time. She felt that she couldn't plan a whole week ahead—her bad days simply knocked her out, so much so that she could not complete even minimal self-care tasks. May Morganson's anticipated but unpredictable bad days, which usurped her life, led her to live almost totally in the present.[5] She did so because living in the present muted and minimized her illness.

Certain bad days lead to a life founded on illness or immersion within it. As such, they occupy the frontier between the borders of intrusive illness and immersion in it.

Spiraling Effects

Intrusive illness has spiraling effects that, in turn, further intrude upon life. Among these effects are the consequences for valued pursuits and self-images and interpersonal relationships.

How and what the illness preempts, when and how long it preempts, and its predicted duration all figure in whatever stance and strategy the ill person takes toward it.

How illness intrudes upon anyone's life affects definitions of it. Persistent, yet relatively invisible, symptoms make it possible to prolong the period before illness preempts valued pursuits and self-images. Six years ago, Tina Reidel kept working despite being in constant pain from arthritis. During this time, she described what her body felt like: "It takes all my concentration just to keep my body going. And I feel like I'm walking around on crushed eggshells and I have to protect my body all the time. . . . You're walking down the street . . . no one can tell. It's real, like a paradox. No one can tell there's anything wrong with you unless they're real perceptive. But you feel like you're just struggling—like each step is just really painful."

Not infrequently, symptoms of an "invisible" illness or of side-effects from medication remain invisible to almost everyone, including those who experience them. Metabolic diseases, renal failure, and steroid treatments may all cause changes in response and mood. For example, Roger Ressmeyer, who has diabetes, writes about insulin shock:

> Severe shock is a frightening, profoundly mind-altering experience. The brain begins to shut down, layer by layer, and unusual personality traits take command. First is a general sensation of nervousness. Next, logic and reason are wiped out of consciousness. Emotion is magnified. Happiness becomes glee, sadness becomes misery, distrust becomes paranoia, anger may become rage. . . . In the middle of an argument with a close friend, I suddenly lost control and landed a punch. I was shocked, horrified. I consider myself a gentle and non-violent person, yet I had clearly become "possessed" by a violent urge. Almost as soon as it happened, I realized that what was "possessing" me was insulin shock and my careening blood sugar. (1983:5)

Ressmeyer identified what was happening to him. Not everyone does. Subsequently, behavior gets pinned to the individual's personality or situation. An older woman believed her difficulty in concentrating was due to the tense office politics at work; much later she discovered that she was having medication side-effects. Until such discovery, further symptoms and medication side-effects can remain unnoted for lengthy periods and, as in Ressmeyer's story, can give rise to startling, unwelcome images of self. When people discover the causes, they feel enormous relief, if regaining control seems possible.

Not surprisingly, visible, unpredictable, and mortifying symptoms cause people to define a loss of control much earlier than those with invisible, but known, symptoms. If embarrassing symptoms are visible but illness is not, people usually curtail their activities sharply. John Garston's uncontrollable coughing riveted attention on him in public. He said, "But it is, you know, it is embarrassing, no matter what—spitting up and all of that. . . . But . . . I guess possibly one of the reasons why I am reclusive is that . . . that's definitely one of them and, you know, it has curtailed social activities, things like that, on my part."

Illness preempts valued pursuits and self-images along three time dimensions: the daily round, the life structure, and the life cycle. I will discuss strategies for handling the daily round in

Chapter 6 and only briefly outline three key points here. First, the relative restrictiveness or flexibility of the daily round shapes whether intrusive illness will preempt someone's usual pursuits. The latitude to fit a daily schedule around illness and regimen allows a person more control over pursuits and self-presentations. A company sales representative who works out of his home enjoys much greater flexibility than a surgical nurse. Second, the time during the day when illness is most intrusive affects whether one can prevent it from preempting valued pursuits and self-images. Several people managed to work because they could control their symptoms until mid-afternoon. Others struggled through an entire workday, then found themselves overcome by fatigue by evening. When they got home, they gave in to illness, after valiantly completing the workday. A number of respondents echoed this woman who said, "I collapse."

Third, narrowed worlds resulted when the daily round consisted only of vital activities, work, and self-care (Brooks and Matson 1987; Fagerhaugh 1975). These men and women could not pursue relationships, hobbies, or recreation. They barely maintained themselves, much less their households. A school nurse with a metabolic condition gave up most activities except her job. She asked, "Where did my evenings go? What did I get done? Three hours pass and I didn't even know where it went. The next day, I wondered what I had done the night before."

The daily round shapes, supports, and solidifies an individual's life structure. The life structure includes activities, daily round, future plans, and the present experience of time. As Levinson (1978) points out, the life structure shifts and changes throughout the life cycle. Though illness prompts changes, in turn, the life structure shapes the extent to which an intrusive illness preempts pursuits. A slow-paced life with few external demands helps to preserve and prolong earlier pursuits; they simply take longer to realize. For some years, several young adults had fluid, rather unstructured, lives. They did not hold regular jobs; nor did they adhere to regular schedules. They preferred pursuits like socializing with friends and forms of self-exploration. They also lacked a finely tuned linear time perspective. Having few time pressures, their lifestyles and time perspectives muted the effect of intrusive symptoms. For example, Sara Shaw had enrolled in college before she first became ill, although she had seldom attended classes. She recalled, "I just laid in bed for days, you know, never going to school; I didn't even show up like for semesters on end . . . I would say that I probably went on my own pacing before that [becoming ill] to some degree. . . . I really didn't worry about the fact that I didn't know whether I got up that day, you know, whether I'd done something a week ago."

Later, when the momentum of these young people's lives increased as they set career goals or had children, they discovered how intrusive their symptoms had become. Having limited time and multiple demands upon it pinpoints attention on functioning. In addition, busy younger people compared themselves and the structure of their lives to age peers rather than to people with similar conditions. When they judged themselves by the standards of people their own age, they almost always fell short. Simultaneously, they sensed a sharpened contrast between health and illness. And, like many Americans, these young people saw health as the norm, something to take for granted, especially when young.

In early midlife, most respondents' lives were structured around jobs and families, and occasionally, school. Their concerns centered on handling their responsibilities and on maintaining their independence. Whether they could maintain a life structure similar to the one that preceded illness often depended upon the amount of social and economic support they could muster. Part of that support translates into access to and coverage for medical care. After his heart attack, Mike Reilly had to borrow money from his brother, and his wife had to become the breadwinner. He said, "And it's [her job] helped us tremendously because—because of their health program. I automatically was covered by Sequoia Health Maintenance Plan and with their coverage for care despite existing conditions. At that time, prescriptions were just killing us."

The structure of elderly people's lives usually differed from younger respondents; also, their expectations differed from younger counterparts.[6] Frequently, their lives muted the visibility of intrusive symptoms. Also, they could gauge what they felt they could accomplish without feeling pressured to do more. One elderly woman commented, "I don't have to get up early anymore, so I often don't. If I wake up stiff and tired, I just stay in bed longer where it's warm and comfortable."

The life structure of elders may not complement that of younger spouses or adult children. Five years ago, at the age of thirty-four, Vera Mueller married Ted McCartney, a retired mechanic and political activist. He had cared for his first wife, Meg, until she died. Since then, his emphysema and cancer had progressed. He said:

> Everybody would say, "Why wouldn't you have Meg put in a home?" It would never come to mind to me to do something like that. If you love somebody, that's it; it doesn't matter. My kids draw similar parallels, and a lot of people do; they say, "Well, why doesn't Vera go to the desert with you; that's where you can breathe." I can also see her point that after I'm gone, she's going to have to be able to work and unless she gets her career going pretty soon, she's not going to be able to do that very well. And so what's best for her career is not best for my breathing.

In contrast, Vera had already told me that Ted was still angry about her not going to the desert and more generally, about how she responded to his illness. She said:

> I think that expectation [of receiving total care] was there. I think in his mind that he expected me to do him the same way [as he had done for Meg], but it's clearly not the same situation. For one thing, his health is better when he has to take care of himself. In other words, he's the kind that he would let me do everything for him; he would become totally an invalid and love every minute of it . . . where he gets upset with me is that I say, "Look you aren't going to be around to take care of me when I'm sixty-five years old . . . and I have to see to it that I can take care of myself." . . . And he gets very mad at me.

Similar tensions arise when isolated aged parents must rely on their adult children who have multiple commitments.

Aged men and women often assumed that they would lead narrowed, even restricted, lives. Moreover, they believed that reasonable people should expect to feel worse as they age. Here again, these elders defined the "appropriateness" of illness in relation to the life cycle. Just before I asked a ninety-one-year-old woman about her chronic illness, she had recited a litany of symptoms. She giggled merrily and replied, "Heavens, dear, I'm not ill; I'm just *old*."

The meanings and priorities preempted by illness also shape an individual's experience and stance toward it. Intrusive symptoms remain less visible when someone does not need to fulfill multiple obligations. Goals, priorities, relationships, and time-frames affect the meaning ill people give to intrusive illness. When a young single woman confronted her potentially life-threatening illness with equanimity, she had no career or special goals, limited family contact, and few close friends. She compared herself to a middle-aged woman who also faced a life-threatening illness but who had a family, career, and goals. Noting this woman's extreme fear of death, the young woman matter-of-factly remarked, "No wonder she is so afraid; she has more to lose than I do." For her, illness did not preempt a valued life at that time.

Similarly, people who have no valued pursuits and few obligations may find intrusive illness less frustrating to cope with than others do. People whose "main" pursuits consisted essentially of side-involvements also had less difficulty dropping them. For example, before they became ill, several students had dropped out of college because of family obligations; they had few regrets about doing this. Later, when their symptoms worsened, they once again left school with little difficulty. As a young woman, Vera Mueller had subordinated her studies to her "hippie" lifestyle. She commented, "Dropping out didn't bother me until I became serious and my education came first." In short, the relative significance of intrusive illness turns, in part, on the structure of ill people's lives.

Both financial and family status influence someone's stance toward illness and shape his or her meanings and priorities concerning it. Financial pressures usually force an ill person to struggle as long as possible to remain working and independent. Financial protection—through spouses, solid pensions, or trust funds—provides a buffer from some of the worst consequences of chronic illness. This protection allows options such as choosing early retirement, moving to a milder climate, or purchasing a car with automatic features. Patricia Kennedy, whose husband was an executive, remarked, "Not everyone can afford to spend thousands on a bathroom or put in a new shower which has a seat in it, you know, or buy a new exercise bike and a whole array of weights. And certainly having money has—made a difference, being able to buy a car that is easier for me to drive made a difference. It would be very difficult to be poor."

Similarly, families provide a buffer for some men and women, which allows them to relinquish obligations. Those who believed that they could rely on family expressed much less anxiety about giving up jobs and other obligations than those without families or who did not wish to rely on them. A single woman felt that she must soon be employable. She stated: "I have to get through [school]. I can't borrow more money or live with Mom forever. Next year I have to be working."

The predicted duration of intrusive illness figures in ill people's stance toward it. Commonly, they develop time-frames—short-term frames for each day and long-term frames for the years ahead. Short-term frames allow them to get through the day.

Many people push themselves through their usual schedule and then attend to their illnesses later. Hence, a lecturer spent his lunch hour on a cot in his office after his morning class. A student forced herself to finish her daily assignments and to organize the family's meals before resting. A businessman handled all his important work in the morning so he could leave the office early in the day. An eligibility worker used flextime so that she could spend afternoons and evenings in bed.

Shorter timeframes allow ill people to maintain their longer timeframes, i.e., their predictions about how much longer they will need to manage intrusive symptoms and struggle to maintain their lives. As Star (1985) observes, they segment uncertainty. Thus, they plan or hope for a definite ending for their current strategy. Hopes of realizing distant plans and dreams provide a greater incentive for struggling to manage arduous daily timeframes than the belief that the present is endless. Hence, the following comments reflect the end in sight:

'til my daughter gets through high school
'til John finishes graduate school and takes over
until next year, then I'm going to go into early retirement

Most of these people believed that they would have better lives after this point in their timeframe. Sometimes they implied that something magical would happen at that point in time. Not only would life become easier, but also their current problems with illness would be ameliorated.

Relationships with others shift and change as ill people's time structure and involvements change. Young children and spouses are closest to and most affected by these changes. Young children may share household work and monitor a parent for symptoms. A spouse's handling of the changes shapes the character of their relationship. Older women, for example, sometimes acted as if their marriage remained the same as it had been before illness, when, in fact, it had changed. Usually an older wife of a sick husband not only gained power in the household, but also over her husband's care, though she may delicately avoid any blatant use of it (Calkins 1970; Lear 1980).

Couples draw apart if illness builds upon their differences. Tina Reidel spent much of her free time with friends, healers, and fellow spiritual seekers. The man with whom she lived worked on his boat or watched sports. She said:

> I spend time with the boyfriend, but we don't seem to get along that well—we have been completely celibate for a couple of years and it's sort of like two cranky people living together, with health problems. And I don't like sports and he likes football. . . . And so I just feel like we sleep in the same bed and I don't even have any contact with him there because my legs hurt so much. It's like he sleeps on his side and he starts snoring, and I say, "Jim, I can't sleep." "What?" "You're snoring." "Well, I got asthma." And it's going on like that.

Intrusive illness often removes the spontaniety from sex. As one woman said, "It takes the romance out of it to have to plan it." Another woman said that her involuntary cries of pain when she moved caused her husband to be reluctant to have sex. A young man said that his new love left him because of his increasing impotence (see also, Kotarba 1983).

Closeness turns on maintaining contact. If contact becomes sporadic, friends and families usually drift apart. Ill people simply may not have the energy to make phone calls, much less to provide companionship or assistance. For example, a middle-aged single woman felt that her once close relationship with her sister had suffered. Earlier, she had done most of the visiting, since she had a car and her sister had children. When she could not drive that distance, nor afford the phone calls, she rarely heard from her sister.

In other instances, relationships falter because people cannot tolerate viewing the ill person's disability or distress. For years, a woman with multiple sclerosis and her brother had shared family outings and holidays. Those shared events dwindled. Her brother told her, "It hurts me so much to see you like this."

Certain relationships thrive on pulling together to combat illness. Some partners find a niche for themselves through the other's illness (Speedling 1982). And they may also enjoy new-found authority in the household. They like feeling useful and involving themselves in care. Lara Cobert described her former boyfriend's sense of loss when she improved:

> In a screaming, yelling battle, he said, "You had it all once. You got sick and I could take care of you. But you went and got well and took it away." It was very interesting to me listening to him say that. He liked it! I always thought of him as *so* powerful. I was scared to death of him, and I'm not usually scared of people. He didn't apparently have much sense of personal power. The only time he was totally comfortable was when I was powerless in one way. . . . I thought it was disgusting.

More commonly, ill people claim more control over resources than others wish them to have. Sometimes ill people assume the right to delegate tasks and to extract extra attention from intimates. Many find, however, that their claims become negotiable and others place tacit, but firm, limits on the amount and kind of attention they will give.

Keeping Illness Contained

What happens as an intrusive illness continues? How do people handle it? Three stances toward illness flow from their degree of acceptance of it and the meanings they attach to it: they either embrace, incorporate, or contain it. Here I focus on keeping illness contained, but first I briefly describe embracing and incorporating it. Embracing illness goes beyond reconciling self to it or accepting it. People welcome it. They take their images of self from it. Illness lends meaning to life and imposes a daily routine. Embracing illness fosters accepting a life founded on it.

Other pursuits and events become subjugated to living with illness. Entire households become restructured. Everyone's emotions revolve on the vissicitudes of illness and on the ill person's moods. By embracing his heart disease, a man controlled his family by constantly reminding them of his impending death. In addition, a foreboding feeling permeated this home.

Although entirely atypical among my respondents, several individuals rather happily adapted to intrusive illness and impairment. A middle-aged man had long been unemployed due to his disabilities. He said candidly, "I'm quite content with things the way they are. I'd hate getting up each day at 6:00 and go through all the bustle and rush of getting through the day. . . . Not for me, thanks. As long as Connie [his wife who had several chronic illnesses and was blind] doesn't get worse, things are just fine."

Only two other individuals seemed satisfied about embracing a life founded on illness. More commonly, people allude to embracing illness and slip into this stance gradually. For them, handling illness provides a raison d'être. While they may disclaim embracing illness, their actions belie their words. Occasionally, a relative suggested that the ill person embraced illness. "You know, she's using it for all the mileage she can get." "He's enjoying the attention." The disparities that relatives noted between the person's expected and actual functioning served as a measure of embracing illness.

Incorporating illness means recognizing it, taking it into account, and living with, rather than for, it. When people incorporate illness, they also are attached to it. However, they build their selves upon illness rather than limit their self-concepts to it. Five years after her lengthy seige with lupus erythematosus, Sara Shaw said, "It's incorporated—it's part of me, but it's a much friendlier part now. We are not at war."

Thus, illness not only becomes a way of identifying self, it becomes a part of self. Lois Jaffe's remarks show how deeply illness can etch self-definition: "Being leukemic is as much a part of my identity as being a woman or being Jewish. It is a part of myself I cannot slough off, no matter how hard I might try" (1977:209).

Many people want to keep their intrusive illness hidden—at least in public, if not also from self; they work at keeping illness contained. They try not to let it rule their lives. They wish to continue at least a semblance of their former lives. Above all, they refuse to rely on their illness as a ready-made excuse for shirking obligations. They may also fear loss and rejection due to stigma. Hence, these people try to keep illness contained through two interrelated strategies: packaging and passing. Packaging means presenting the self so that illness remains contained, separate from the public, and usually, the private self. Passing means functioning without detection of either the illness or its effects.

By packaging illness, a person treats illness as if it is controlled, delimited, and confined to specific realms, such as private life. Packaging means "guarantees" that the illness will not seep out of its containers unexpectedly. Packaging also means that ill people present the self as if it were in control of their illness package. They keep illness tightly wrapped. A conception of illness as external to the self frequently underlies these views. Yet these views also assume that illness can intrude upon the self or perhaps, if improperly contained, take over the self.

When attempting to package illness, people treat outbreaks of their illness as unrelated episodes and hospitalizations as independent units of time. Past events remain distant from present self and unconnected with current health. Each episode, each hospitalization, becomes a separate package, a finished, completed product, not a continuing illness. Ill people may dredge up these past packages and use them as interesting stories, but close them again in order that the contents do not rip open, leak out, or spill into their lives.

Conceptual packaging shapes meanings of illness. How people think about and categorize their illness reflects how they treat it. They may not define their physical status as illness. If anything, it is a "condition." To them, adopting the term "illness" means being sick, allowing closer surveillance by medical professionals and, moreover, sometimes adopting the patient role. Many people see themselves as relatively healthy, except perhaps for delimited symptoms (Bury 1988). For these people, "illness" connotes serious, incapacitating, current symptoms. Hence, a woman felt appalled when a friend referred her to me for my study of chronic illness, although she had had cancer and still suffered from disabling rheumatoid arthritis. For her, cancer, not arthritis, merited the status of a bona fide "illness." And, she avowed that she was cured. Compared to cancer, she saw arthritis as inconsequential. She stated that its effects were "negligible," despite several delicate surgeries, risky treatments, and, formerly, an inability to walk.

By not defining illness, people try to separate it from their lives and to detach it from their self-concepts. Seven years ago, when I asked Vera Mueller about her illness, she responded, "Well, in the first place, I don't see it as an illness. At the very best, it is a condition—or at the very *most*, I should say, a condition. Separate? Oh, I wish it were. It used to be separate from my life; it used to be something that only when other people forced me to, I'd pay attention to, or only when I pushed myself too far, I'd pay attention to."

Shortly thereafter, Vera stated emphatically, "I don't want to be a sick person." She avoided adopting that identity by conceptually ruling out illness. Similarly, the elderly woman who saw herself as old, not ill, then said that for a woman her age, she was exceptionally "well." Taken-for-granted conceptions of aging as deterioration allow for similar conceptual camouflaging. "Aging" reduces incentive for remaining active and provides a ready-made conceptual package to account for growing infirmity. At fifty-eight, Marty Gordon observed, "It's hard to tell what is just aging and what might be connected to the illness."

Family, friends, and professionals sometimes provide the conceptual camouflaging. For years, an elderly woman accepted her doctor's category of "a minor heart murmur." In contrast, another elderly woman with the same type of murmur saw herself as having a disabling heart condition. Paradoxically perhaps, those who incorporate illness occasionally no longer define themselves as "ill" or their conditions as "illness." After having no serious episodes for five years, Sara Shaw remarked, "I tend to think of it [lupus erythematosus] as part of my life, not an illness."

As Vera Mueller's comments above suggest, terms like "condition" or "syndrome" also provide conceptual packages. Ambiguous terms result in varied conceptual packages. For fourteen years—until she had a major episode of multiple sclerosis—Harriet Binetti accepted her neurologist's label that she had "a minor neurological condition." When people asked, "Why are you limping?" or when she wondered, "Why am I so tired?," she explained and discounted her symptoms by saying, "I have a minor neurological condition." How ill people interpret and conceptualize their medical status may either minimize or magnify it.

Self-presentation, which shades into passing, is another major part of packaging (cf. Goffman 1959; Morgan 1982). Younger people, particularly, talked about their appearances. Patricia Kennedy said, "I never go anywhere if I don't feel good. If I don't look good, I just won't go." Vera Mueller exclaimed, "Look at me—I don't look sick; I don't act sick; I often don't feel sick. Whoever would suspect it? I don't want people to know." Concern with appearance turned on keeping illness contained, controlling it, and passing.

Passing entails concealing illness, maintaining a conventional self-presentation, and performing like unimpaired peers (Strauss and Glaser 1975). People attempt to pass for two reasons. First, illness could count against them, or they believe it would (MacDonald 1988; Scambler and Hopkins 1988; Schneider and Conrad 1980; 1983). For example, a business executive thought that knowledge of his illness would put him at a disadvantage in contract negotiations. So he told no one and concealed evidence of it. Second, illness could bring people special privileges because of pity, or possibly, concern.

Passing depends on concealing infirmity. If others know the diagnosis, ill people may acknowledge it but hide its implications. Crises vitiate passing. Visible symptoms such as slurred speech, an unsteady gait, or shortness of breath undermine it (Pinder 1988). An abstract discussion of a person's diagnosis is one thing; exposing infirmity is quite another. Lin Bell's friends knew that she had a heart condition. However, they did not know what would overtax her. She said:

> You learn how to hide infirmities. And mine doesn't show. . . . I'm having company this weekend . . . and they know, you know, that I can't do, but I don't want them doing everything for me, so I bought three gallons of wine. . . . So I bring it to the bottom of the stairs; I stand there for two or three minutes, then I lift each bag up and I lift them up about four stairs and then I follow them up. . . . It takes me fifteen or twenty minutes to get groceries up [to her second floor apartment], but I don't want anybody to know. I mean, if they're out there watching me, they're going to know.

Passing is risky. Obviously, passing depends on competent performances at crucial times and places. Successful passing often requires an alert assistant. A woman's mother monitored her behavior and symptoms at social events. Then, they could leave before the point that her incoordination and slurred speech belied her attempts to pass. A wife covered phone calls for her husband when he experienced confusion. A small boy staked out public places to find locations where his mother could sit or lean. A teenager waited in grocery lines for his mother since she risked losing her balance while standing still.

Passing and packaging permit people to choose how to deal with their illnesses. Paradoxically, however, the very reasons for keeping illness contained—to pursue a career, to keep a job, to develop a relationship—can foster the condtions in which intrusiveness of illness escalates. For example, as Ressmeyer (1983) found, irregular hours, lack of sleep, and fast foods caused havoc with his diabetes, even though he passed for months. In short, risky strategies for keeping illness contained can result in magnifying it and having it flood identity.

Beyond being strategies to maintain self-presentation, passing and packaging also are strategies to preserve self. Containing illness in tight packages and managing to pass alleviates the necessity of facing illness directly. If regimen and symptom control work, someone can deal with illness in small doses. That is, the person reveals illness in controlled gradients to self as well as to others. Thus, thudding realizations about what life might become are avoided. Simultaneously, the person affirms that illness is only what he or she experiences now.

If people can control symptoms and create manageable lives, or if illness remains relatively quiescent, passing and packaging can become taken-for-granted strategies—so much so that these people may believe that their illness is over. But when regimens fail, or the disease flares again, these individuals plummet into depths of self-blame. They believe that they have not done enough. In short, effective packaging and passing strategies encourage redefining illness. And that redefinition sets the stage for dramatic self-blame if the strategies later fail.

Developing a Dialectical Self

The dialectical self is the contrast between the sick or physical self and the monitoring self. Keeping illness contained by impeding progression of illness, rather than merely hiding it, leads to developing a monitoring self. Developing a dialectical self means gaining a heightened awareness of one's body. People who do so believe that they perceive nuances of physical changes. By his second transplant, for example, Mark Reinertsen felt that he had learned to perceive the first signs of organ rejection.

When these people no longer view themselves as "sick," they still monitor their physical selves to save themselves from further illness. Sara Shaw explained that she spent months of "learning time" to be able to discover what her body "needed" and how to handle those needs. She commented, "I got to know it [her ill body]; I got to understand it, and it was just me and mixed connective tissue disease [her diagnosis changed], you know, and I got to respect it and I got to know—to have a real good feeling for time elements and for what my body was doing, how my body was feeling." When I asked her what she meant by "time elements," she replied:

> There's times during the month, during the course of a month, when I'm much more susceptible, and I can feel it. I can wake up in the morning and I can feel it. . . . So I really learned what I was capable of and when I had to stop, when I had to slow down. And I learned to like—give and take with that. And I think that's all programmed in my mind now, and I don't even have to think about it now, you know; I'll know. I'll know when, no matter what's going on, I've gotta go sit down . . . and take it easy . . . that's a requirement of that day. And so consequently, I really don't get sick.

In the dialectical self, the monitoring self externalizes the internal messages from the physical self and makes them concrete. It is as if dialogue and negotiation with ultimate validation of the physical self take place. For example, Mark Reinertsen engaged in "person to kidney" talks to encourage the new kidney to remain with him (see also McGuire and Kantor 1987). A competent monitoring self attends to messages from the physical self, and over time, as Sara Shaw's comment suggests, monitoring becomes taken for granted.

In many ways, the dialectical self is analogous to the dialogue that Mead (1934) describes between the "I" and the "me." The "me" monitors and attends to the "I" that creates, experiences, and feels. The monitoring "me" defines the "I's" behaviors, feelings, impulses, and sensations. It evaluates them and plans action to meet defined needs. Here, an ill person takes his or her physical self as an object, appraises it, and compares it with past physical selves, with perceived health statuses of others, with ideals of physical or mental well-being, with signals of potential crises, and so forth (cf. Gadow 1982).

The dialectical self is one of ill people's multiple selves that emerges in the face of uncertainty. Whether ill people give the dialectical self validity significantly affects their actions. For someone like Sara Shaw, the dialectical self provided guidelines for organizing time, for taking jobs, and for developing relationships with others. With jobs, she believed that she had to guard herself from the stress of too many demands. With friends, she felt she had to place her needs first. With physicians, she resisted their control since she trusted her knowledge about her condition more than theirs.

Practitioners may encourage a monitoring self when it seems to "work," yet condemn it when unsuccessful, or when monitoring tactics conflict with their advice (cf. Kleinman 1988). The development of the dialectical self illuminates the active stance that some people take toward their illnesses and their lives. In short, the dialectical self helps people to keep illness in the background of their lives.

4

Immersion in Illness

The MS [multiple sclerosis], it affects your balance and it affects your bladder and—and I do have a catheter. . . . My stomach is bad. And—and unfortunately, those are areas that really hurt you when you're in a wheelchair.

So there's always a bladder infection. . . . When I came out [from the nursing home], it seems like that's all I deal with—bladder infections. . . . So I just cleared a bladder infection. It was stressful and it's just been a year of that bladder infection and I probably have another one and this has just been a week and a half. So I can always tell with my back pain and the way I sleep and—and with every bladder infection, the medicines—they kill the good bacteria, too. So you get a yeast infection and it's like you just live around the clock [with illness and care] and it's—and that's—if all I have to deal with, that's one thing, but I have all the stress of my—my family. And that's taken a real toll. And then my bowels don't work. This bladder medicine gives you diarrhea.

Medications. Regimens. Setbacks. Suffering. At forty-five, Harriet Binetti constantly attended to acute conditions that disrupted and even threatened her life. Relentless pain and mounting troubles stretched minutes into hours. During the past decade, Harriet's health had rapidly deteriorated. Initially, multiple sclerosis had left her with minor disabilities and some inconvenience. By the time we first met, Harriet could only move her head.

Harriet Binetti frequently became immersed in unpredictable, devastating flare-ups or acute conditions. She needed contradictory medications for different complications and had drug allergies besides. Medi-Cal insurance did not readily cover the

73

substitute medications that she could tolerate. Trying to balance her symptoms, medications, and treatments without making her sicker and poorer resembled putting together an intricate and engrossing puzzle—a puzzle that devoured time and demanded attention.

Nonetheless, Harriet Binetti tried to have a life beyond illness. When she could, she attended community events in her electric wheelchair. Low-income housing, Medi-Cal insurance, and attendant care allowed her to live autonomously on a limited disability benefit.

Before she obtained low-income housing and attendant care, Harriet had spent three long years in nursing homes with virtually no control over her life. As a result, illness and death frightened her less than the prospect of going to another nursing home. She took refuge in the pleasant apartment that she shared with Sally, a young friend who served as her nursing attendant.

Harriet Binetti's congenial bond with Sally contrasted sharply with the tension and torment in her relationships with her adult children. These relationships, too, shaded her experience of illness. Her daughter's marriage to a recovering drug addict disappointed her, as did her son's perpetual unemployment and sporadic tangles with the police. She and her daughter, Susan, had had a row when Harriet discovered that Susan had smoked marijuana throughout her recent pregnancy. Though Harriet apologized for not handling her feelings well, she had not heard from Susan since. Harriet's longstanding tensions with her son, Robert, erupted shortly thereafter. Although Harriet had few financial and social resources with which to put a life together, Robert continued to ask her for financial help and for emotional support. She told me that she said to him: " 'I didn't ask to be put into this chair [wheelchair] and it's enough for me to take care of myself, and I think I do fairly well for being disabled. And I can't understand why you, as a normal human being can't do half as well as I can. Not you, Robert. I can't—I can't.' "

Harriet believed that her ex-husband and children blamed Robert's troubles, including having the AIDS virus, on her. When I asked, "You?" She said, "Yeah, because I had to get married [to Robert's father] and because I had to get married, his father wasn't very good to Robert . . . and well, Robert didn't find that out until this year. . . . And you know, talk about nailing Jesus Christ to the cross—I—He didn't suffer half as much as I got nailed for. I mean . . . for getting pregnant before I got married."

The ripples of the past absorbed Harriet Binetti's thoughts, and the ravages of multiple sclerosis flooded her days. Yet she did not passively succumb to illness. Despite her medical, family, and financial problems, Harriet tried to have a good life. Both Harriet and Sally created numerous innovations to manage Harriet's care more easily and to grant her more autonomy. They improvised a way for her to use her speaker phone without having help. Harriet devised a way to drink water independently by attaching a jug with tubes to her wheelchair. They both kept abreast of legal changes that might offer Harriet increased services. And they both showed amazing resourcefulness in finding and using community agencies and programs.

After the three years in nursing homes, Harriet relished her independence and valued her friendship with Sally. Time took on new meaning. Certainly, illness, pain, and perplexing troubles sometimes engulfed her in unending time. And the routines of care shaped her days. Such immersion can separate anyone from the rhythms of ordinary adult life. Subsequently, the temporal order of immersion in illness leads one into an extraordinary reality with its own structure and rules.

However, like most ill people, Harriet Binetti tried to limit being immersed in illness. When her physical condition stabilized, Harriet's and Sally's interests in cooking, outings, and discussing current events broke the illness routines. Harriet's interests kept her grounded in conventional realities and ordinary pursuits. Like others, Harriet resisted becoming immersed in illness, although her life was founded upon it. When people have choices and resources, they can move back and forth between immersion in illness and having a life founded upon it.

In either case, illness refocuses one's time perspective. Time seems revised and reshaped. In turn, changes in viewing and experiencing time may lead to changes in self-concept.

A Life Founded upon Illness

Many people, like Harriet Binetti, try to carry on ordinary but limited pursuits although their lives have become founded upon illness. They try to keep illness in the background, the backdrop on which daily scenes are played (Lewis 1985; Pitzele 1985; Register 1987). They still take the external world as their point of reference, despite the encroachments illness has made upon them. Although illness *orders* life, it does not entirely define or fill it; people attend to other things as well for months or, intermittently, for years. They raise children; they keep house; they maintain self-care. They may even work occasionally when they can, or serve as volunteers.

When life becomes founded on illness, illness is not simply intrusive. No longer can people add illness to the structure of their lives; instead, they must *reconstruct* their lives upon illness. Hence, they cannot simply add regimens, rest periods, timeouts, and so forth to work, school, leisure, and family activities. The requirements of illness and health come first and now define their pursuits.

A life founded upon illness lies a hair above immersion in it. Health remains precarious; crises, complications, and setbacks often force people into immersion. Afterwards, they might again have a restricted life founded on illness. At that point, illness again partially recedes into the background of daily life. As debilitating episodes increase, having a life founded upon illness may be the most that a person can hope for.

Most of these people don't work.[1] They can't. Ann Rorty's unsuccessful back surgery, bowel incontinence, and heart disease forced her to quit her job. She reiterated what her surgeon had said: "He said that definitely, I can't go back and do the job I was doing. No lifting. . . . For three years straight, I was . . . lifting maybe eleven buckets of grease a night. . . . I was carrying it out to the back, two buckets to dump and I finally weighed them, when I was getting ready to have this surgery this last time, just before my last day at work, I weighed the buckets and they were nineteen pounds and that's quite a bit to be lifting from the floor up, you know, that many times a night."

When a "physical" condition affects mental functioning, or mental strain reduces usual productivity, ill people are forced to leave work. Though they may handle household tasks quite well, they feel confused, unable to concentrate, and immobilized by distractions, which interfere with their work. A former attorney stated:

> I don't have problems concentrating—I have problems *shifting* my concentration from one area to another. So if I have to think about the source of a legal process as it was in 1870, 1887 or something . . . I can use my mind like a search light—bring my mind to bear on some of these, you know, fundamental concepts, but if I have to remember to put the staple in the letter and then turn the typewriter off and punch the—you know, and do a number of different, simple little things, I can't do it. I can't do it.

A few people still manage to do limited work when they could control the structuring, scheduling, pacing, and content of their work. Retired executives sometimes did intermittent consulting for their businesses. Harry Bauer's heart condition caused his early retirement from his powerful union office ten years ago, but the union "kind of created a special thing to let me work as much as I wanted to work when I first retired."

For those without an adequate income, a life founded upon illness means work—hard work. Limited money, reduced access to services, insurance problems, and enormous hurdles to obtain a disability benefit all mean work. Lifestyles change drastically with less income, more bills, and new needs. If no advocates help, ill people must do the work themselves despite being physically depleted. When she was forty-seven, Nancy Swenson had constant disturbing symptoms. Also, she was in the midst of completing massive amounts of eligibility documentation for a disability benefit for herself and for services for her mother. She described how her condition intervened with preparing her applications:

> When I have bad nights with that [sleep apnea], I'm just so physically exhausted that it seems like . . . there's just not enough time because I can't get going. Or on the other hand,

when I'm like that, I get behind and then when I feel good, I have to catch up on back stuff and try to get caught up and get a little ahead so that if I'm down again I won't have to feel the pressures of, "Oh, God, I'm just sitting here and I have all this to do."

I asked, "What sorts of things play on your mind that you need to do?" She said:

> *Paperwork.*
> I spent two years fighting for my Social Security and did all of my paperwork, with Ed's [disability rights advocate] help. Social Services, they give me three social workers. One for food stamps, one for Medi-Cal, and one for General Assistance. All three of them—not them—the computers—whatever, have messed up. So the paperwork is incredible that they send me to keep up. Well, then I have my mother's [who has Alzheimer's] paperwork along with my own paperwork to try to do, which is . . . an *absolute* impossibility to do in my mom's waking hours or my mom's time in this house.

The work extends to other people and exhausts resources. Patricia Kennedy's husband interceded with her employer about her insurance coverage when she had to stop working. Not only was Bonnie Presley's health depleted, but also, she went through an inheritance for doctor bills and living expenses when she could not work and did not have insurance. She even had to sign her car over to her landlord to cover three months of late rent. Afterwards, she only had the meager support of General Assistance. Bargaining to cover expenses was work. Getting information about getting help was work. Traveling fifty miles to attend workshops to assist her in applying for a disability benefit proved too exhausting.

Nevertheless, a life founded on illness can have rewards. Nancy Swenson said, "I can't do the things that I used to be able to do, but see if you can't, you don't dwell on that, you go on and you find the things that you can enjoy. . . . I think [ill people] do fine if you socialize. [Then] you don't dwell upon your illness."

Experiencing Immersion

As people become immersed in illness, the structure of their lives changes and immediate concerns inundate them. Priorities change.

Recasting Life

Illness keeps shooting into the foreground. The momentum and impact of illness recast people's lives into new forms. Sara Shaw said, "It [illness] was my life. It wasn't part of my life; it *was* my life." Try as they will, these people cannot bring themselves out of illness; it overtakes them. Mark Reinertsen remarked, "The last six months or so, it's been one thing after another. My hemocrit's down, [I'm] vomiting blood. Last week I had real trouble breathing—my weight went down, but my fluid level went up. . . . I've been feeling emotionally overloaded with my [disrupted] plans, my stuff [continuous complications], helping my friends with their stuff [problems]."

After years of valiantly dealing with his condition, Mark Reinertsen offered these comments as observed facts. But for others, a pervading sense of victimization accompanies immersion in illness. Illness and disability stay in the foreground—ever present and ever vexing. For such people, illness and disability affront self. Beliefs that life would be perpetually positive, progressive, and productive promise control over one's self, one's life, and one's fate. Yet these people had become ill. To them, their illness means more than an insult to the body; it represents an unwarranted, illegitimate attack upon the self.[2] Their despair over not recovering floods their self-concepts and subsequently, sinks them deeper into immersion in illness. For them, illness has recast their self-concepts as well as their bodies and lives.

With these feelings, continuing immersion raises questions about whether to live at all. For example, Ron Rosato's rapid downhill course of multiple sclerosis led him to a suicide attempt:

When I first got this problem, it was almost instantly—I got into drugs because I wanted out of this life. I saw this life [with multiple sclerosis] and I couldn't handle it, you know. And I did drugs and I did everything I could to end it. And it just wouldn't happen. About six years ago, I was doing freebase and I was arced [drugged out of his mind]. And then, God, I thought that was it. I had to be strapped in bed. And I just said, "Lord, please let me go tonight." And I fell asleep and I woke up in the morning; man was I pissed off. Oh, was I pissed off.

Facing Dependency

Immersion in illness means experiencing the vulnerability of one's body: facing dependency. Certainly physical dependency, if not also social and economic dependency, can result from illness. However, many ill people just glance at their dependency and turn away. They cannot accept it, even when foisted upon them. For them, dependency remains a greater specter than death.

At this point, ill people may reject anything that they view as a symbol of failing health or as a testimony to dependency. Goldie Johnson's inexplicably rapid progression of emphysema and heart disease made walking impossible. She said, "I turned down the wheelchair twice. Before, I'd go 'ugh'. . . . That's the hardest thing about being a shut-in—you've been on the go all your life, then [to] be a shut-in. . . . I had a total heart attack and emphysema and that put me in the wheelchair."

Married people often assume that their spouses will serve as their arms and legs to do many tasks that are now difficult or impossible. However, even in long-term happy marriages, dependency alters and strains relations. Robert F. Murphy's benign spinal cord tumor caused paralysis of his arms and legs. He states:

During the course of a day, I usually ask Yolanda [his wife] for dozens of small services, over and above the main care she gives me. Since I know she is overburdened, I generally hesitate to ask for things and feel slightly guilty about bothering her—a guilt that becomes added to that caused by my damaged body. As a result, I am especially sensitive to the tone of her response. Do I detect a note of impatience? Is she annoyed? Is she overtired? Should I have asked her? Does that slight inflection say, "What the hell does he want from me now?" (1987:213–214)

The prospect of dependency poses horrendous problems for single people. When Bonnie Presley was sick, broke, and unable to function, she saw only two alternatives—go on disability or get married. She recounted telling the eligibility worker:

I said, "I don't want to do this [marry Ken]." I said, "I need to be independent; I need to be able—I've been forced into marriages all my life and I feel like I'm going to be forced into something again. Go live with a man."
[To me]: I don't mind crawling up there in that bed by myself right now. I hurt, you know and I don't feel sexy—just the thought of kissing me [shakes head in disinterest]. . . . [with fear and fervor] I hope I *don't* have to marry Ken just to survive. I don't want to be forced into a relationship just to keep from starving.

And what happens when people have no one? The specter of dependency means silence or institutionalization. Subsequently, these people face dependency and handle it by eliminating chunks of their lives, even at risk to their health (see Chapter 6). Others face dependency by accepting poor care and great loneliness rather than asking for help, for comfort, for love.

Pulling In

Immersion in illness shrinks social worlds. It forces people to pull into their inner circle while pulling away from others. They must try to protect themselves and to keep some control over their lives. They have little strength for anything beyond illness. Pulling in begins with crisis or intrusive illness and gains momentum with immersion. Typically, pulling in is a taken-for-granted adaptation to serious illness. Pulling in permits ill people and their caregivers to tighten the boundaries of their lives, to reorder their priorities, and to struggle with the exigencies of illness.

Usually, people tighten their essential relationships and loosen problematic bonds and casual ties. For example, a young woman temporarily pulled away from her mother and siblings with whom she had tense relationships. Simultaneously, she reaffirmed the bonds with her husband and children. She felt that she could not afford the time, physical energy, and psychic space to handle anything more. Hence, she took a timeout from her mother and siblings while struggling with illness.

Certainly pulling in allows for ranking relationships and making priorities, which can occur by default. In retrospect, people sometimes discover that pulling in lets them jettison difficult people from their lives.

Ordinary life cycle transitions may coincide with and intensify pulling in. Like everyone, ill people have parents who die, children with troubles, spouses with midlife crises, and partners who retire. Furthermore, by pulling in for illness, people have fewer social resources to draw upon during their own predictable life cycle transitions. Although necessary, pulling in to handle serious illness sets an empty stage for future social isolation.

Slipping into Illness Routines

Many people slip into consuming illness routines by: 1) experiencing devastating symptoms that preclude other involvements, 2) requiring maintenance care, 3) ordering the day around illness and regimen, and 4) ceasing to look beyond illness and care to view and to form their lives. Life echoes that within institutions; the routines of care shape each day.

Being immersed in illness routines involves continued separation from conventional life, prolonged immobility, and unchanging time. Conventional life and earlier pursuits recede from the present and fade into the past. Life consists of the repetitive routines of managing illness. For example, seriously ill dialysis patients must structure their lives around the rhythms of having dialysis three days a week. Also, these patients must adapt to their bodily rhythms during each day on dialysis and each day off dialysis. Those rhythms seldom blend. May Morganson slipped into illness routines after her forced retirement from work due to kidney failure. She described her days:

> And it seems like I don't really have that much spare time. It's really surprising. . . . Sometimes dialysis is not [does not go] very well, sometimes I'll come home feeling pretty bum. And sometimes the next day it's not too good.
>   . . . [Dialysis] just about takes up the day. . . . I'm supposed to be on at 12:30, but sometimes then don't get on until 1:00, then I'm dialyzed for four and a half hours and then it takes approximately half an hour to be taken off the machine and to have it clot. So quite often it's 6:00 or 6:30 before I ever leave there. So the day is shot—
>   . . . If I am not feeling very well, I'll stop at my daughter's for half an hour or so and just rest, you know, sort of 'til I feel better, and then I'll come on home.

Like many ill people, May Morganson limited her activities so that she could get to dialysis and maintain herself no matter how she felt. She also planned a few days ahead so that she could rest during a terrible day. Identifying the symptoms or procedures that cause further incapacitation helps to keep illness routine. May could anticipate the ill-effects of having a blood transfusion. She remarked, "I just sort of think, 'Well, now, I'm getting a blood transfusion today, I'd better plan on not doing much of anything tomorrow.' And that's usually the way it works."

May Morganson had to think about how to manage her routine because she lived alone. However, the routine can also determine the day of a caregiver, or of an entire family, if there is one (Corbin and Strauss 1988; Strong 1988).

What happens when someone becomes immersed in illness? Pursuits narrow and shrink. Boundaries of experience contract. Control over time lessens. Though the extent of disability can contribute to these shrinking boundaries, the social context has greater significance. Like Harriet Binetti, Ron Rosato had attendant care after being in and out of nursing homes. He could not feed himself or read, but he did watch TV "because there is nothing else to do." Although he had a kind attendant, Ron had neither the intellectual stimulation nor the access to events and activities that Harriet had. He possessed little control over his life, while Harriet Binetti enjoyed considerable autonomy. Ron had a room in his attendant's home; in contrast, Harriet had her own apartment. Ron compared his past pursuits with his present immobility: "I used to write a lot of poetry and I used to do art work, and I used to sing and write music and play the harmonica. And all that stuff is nil now. It's not around. So what do I do? Lie in bed. That's all I can do."

When an individual feels confined in a shrunken world, with few opportunities to create a self, he or she will remain acutely aware of the loss of self and may rail against it. Although Ron Rosato viewed being in the board and care home as "1,000 degrees better than a nursing home," he still lacked control over his life and his care. During the past few years, he had been buffetted from nursing home to acute hospital to nursing home. Having these changes imposed upon him underscored his lack of autonomy. When I asked him, "How has it been for you to make these changes?" he said, "Well, I don't like it, but . . . I have no choice. And there again, that was my reasoning for wanting to get out [of life]. And I think it's good reasoning."

The boundaries that someone's physical condition imposes restrict social life and, hence, can limit the sense of self. In addition, physical and financial dependence evoke pejorative labels, further constricting the boundaries of the self. And the longer the boundaries of the self remain limited, the more repetitive life becomes. Similarly, as illness continues, most people lose ways of shaping and giving meaning to their days.

The television set connects many ill people to the world and programs their day. Gloria Krause described the two years of recuperating from multiple surgeries and radiation: "But I didn't do much. I didn't do much socializing or anything. For two years, I watched TV. I'd watch Johnny Carson every night. I was a real nightowl—I'd sleep in, then I'd get up by 11:30 or 12:30 and I'd watch TV. I was a pro. I'd watch Tom Snyder; he came on after Johnny Carson. I studied these people and I'd know every move Johnny was going to do."

Of course, the rhythm and structure provided by television programs can precede immersion in illness. For example, a number of elderly people have long been wedded to their television programs. Years later, they fill their days with the restrictions imposed by illness and the incentives offered by television. Seventy-eight year-old Bessie Thompkins fit an interview with me in between her noon soap opera and afternoon game show. When I asked her what an ordinary day was like, she said:

> I sit here.
> [She elaborated matter of factly.] I generally get up between 8:00 and 8:30. There's nothing to get up for. On a regular day, I have my breakfast, water my flowers, and take care of my plants and stuff. I do my dish and spoon that I have. I don't do any housework around here; Stella [home health aide] does it all. She gets paid for it so why should I do it? [Laughs.] I have some African violets that I planted from seeds growing. I pick up last night's paper and I read that. I watch TV, my regular programs, then at 12:00, I shut it off and fix my lunch [a serving of cottage cheese]. Then at 12:30, I watch "As the World Turns."

When illness so limits life and steadily progresses, most people—like Ron Rosato, May Morganson, and Bessie Thompkins—find that their worlds shrink. But others like Harriet Binetti and Nancy Swenson move between immersion and a life founded on illness. Subsequently, they still retain ties to conventional life. Because their separation from conventional life remains episodic and partial, rather than continuous and complete, their worlds shrink more slowly.

Weathering a Serious Episode

A serious episode consumes life. Health deteriorates and flare-ups get worse. Weathering a serious episode means suffering through the upheavals of a progressive, unpredictable illness. This immersion resembles having a devastating acute illness, only it lasts—and lasts. And recovery? Rather than hope for total recovery, ill people just hope to regain limited functioning. Though illness may not threaten life immediately, additional crises and possible death lie around every corner.

The vantage point for viewing immersion in a serious episode shapes its direction. When comparing a serious episode with the boundaries and plateaus of immersion in routines, the course of illness plunges downward. When compared to a crisis, the course of illness creeps upward. The patient might live. Still, his or her condition remains serious and the prognosis risky. In short, immersion in a serious episode lies between slipping into routines and being in crisis.

Nowadays, extremely ill people languish within lengthy serious episodes. Many elderly people and people with limited insurance find themselves dangling an inch above crisis yet still immersed in illness. Twenty years ago, if they had lived at all, they would have remained in the hospital. Now, hospitals send them home. Here, the organization of care shapes medical definitions of patients' conditions and decisions about how to handle them.

Even if the crisis has "passed" and is in the past, residuals of it create or compound the present immersion. Under these conditions, ill people must cope with more; simultaneously, they have less wherewithal with which to cope. The present overwhelms them. The future looks worse. The threat of another crisis or death remains. After a sixty-two-year-old woman had been discharged from the hospital, she reflected upon her multiple medical crises: "I guess they are small strokes, but I don't know, everytime it happens, there's less of me left."

Steady changes and constant setbacks shatter regimens and rupture routines. Neither ill people nor their caregivers can control their symptoms. Moreover, ill people may feel that they cannot control their response to them. A young woman with severe dermatitis and colitis said: "At that moment when you're alone in your room, the itching is so bad you want to claw your skin off or the pain is so bad . . . with colitis, [I'm] crying, sitting on a toilet or just curling up in a ball in bed and covering up my head and crying, crying. There was nothing I could do. I just had great pain. I was out of control. My body was taken over at that point."

Being captured and confined by a tormented body renders one powerless. A middle-aged man's cancer and subsequent surgeries kept him in constant pain. No longer could he oversee the household affairs. Nor could he even attend to his youngest son's play-by-play recitation of the exploits of the basketball team for which he had served as assistant coach. His pain drew him into himself and his immediate experience of it. He lamented, "This [his illness] is awful; this is just disgusting. I can't concentrate on anything [except the pain], can't get anything done. All I do is move from the chair to the couch and back again when it hurts too much. I can't even sleep in a bed anymore; it's just too painful. There's nothing I can do to ease the pain."

As illness overtakes people, they lose the identifications from the past; those, too, are swept away. Patricia Kennedy had derived much pride from being a wife, supermom, community volunteer, and churchworker. She said, "[I recognized] that I would no longer be able to do the things that I was involved in, particularly the volunteer activities, which I have enjoyed, you know, working well with kids and the liturgy work that I was doing. I had lost . . . that identification of self—for right after the diagnosis I was so ill that I had lost it—temporarily even the parent, even the *wife* to a certain degree."

Time in Immersion and Immersion in Time

During illness, time takes on new dimensions and meanings. Chief among these is the feeling of becoming lost in time as well as in illness. Further, different meanings of time emerge depending on whether someone experiences a routine or serious immersion in illness.

Unchanging Time

An immersion in routines leads to a sense of unchanging time (Calkins 1970). The same set of experiences is repeated with little variation; time seems static. The day moves in a cycle reproducing yesterday—and all the yesterdays before. The illness and treatment regimen changes slowly, if at all.[3] Sourkes (1982:55) describes a "sense of being suspended in space and time, without defined movement in either direction."[4] Thomas Mann captures the essence of unchanging time in *The Magic Mountain:*

> For the moment we need only recall the swift flight of time— even of quite a considerable period of time—which we spend in bed when we are ill. All the days are nothing, but the same day repeating itself—or rather, since it is always the same day, it is incorrect to speak of repetition, a continuous present, an identity, an everlastingness—such words as these would better convey the idea. . . . You are losing a sense of the demarcations of time, that its units are running together disappearing, and what is being revealed to you as the true content of time is merely a dimensionless present in which they bring you broth. (1924:183– 184)

Certainly, scant daily contact with few individuals contributes to a sense of unchanging time. Also, if those few people merely expedite the routines of care, then their presence likely adds to the patient's sense of unchanging time.

Days slip by. The same day keeps slipping by. Durations of time lengthen since few events break up the day, week, or month. Illness seems like one long uninterrupted duration of time. A young woman recalled her four-year bout of colitis: "So a lot of—so my life just continued to stay the same. So I was sick and I had the same dead-end job and yeah, it's all the same. That felt very like nothing changed. So what's time when nothing changes? It was slow then."

Most likely, the sameness of this woman's job magnified the sameness of her illness.[5] For her, as well as for others, all her endeavors melded into one long undifferentiated event. Sara Shaw recalled that during the year she was incapacitated,

> I lost all track of time that whole year. I didn't have a good concept of time. I didn't know what day it was. . . . The whole

year passed that way. When I think back to that year, it's like one feeling. You know, when you are well, you're changing moods all the time. But when I was sick, it was one feeling for an entire year. I can snap back into that feeling of that year and its the same thing. So to me it's like I could have been in bed.

Sara described the even unchanging time as "monochromatic time," a time that flowed without dimension, change, or color; "it was all the same shade of gray." She added, "[Time] was definitely different than any way I had experienced time in my life. And it was like a fog, you know, like having a fog around me. And there were no real things to set it off. . . . There weren't any markers."

An elderly man who lived in a board and care institution described time as "endless boredom." For him, the institutional rituals, gossip, and tensions scarcely punctured that boredom or punctuated time. Instead, time slipped away without meaning.

A lengthy hospitalization without improvement or decline fosters slipping into routines. Hospital patients, too, found that the stretched quality of unchanging time engulfed them in a sea of dimensionless time, an ever-lengthening present (Mann 1924). Mark Reinertsen described the blurring of time during his lengthy hospitalization when he experienced transplant rejection:

Oh time passes forever. Takes forever to—yeah—I never never—if it hadn't been for my transplant book, which you keep, and you keep daily . . . I wouldn't have known what day it was. And when I'd get to the end of the month and I didn't know if there were thirty or thirty-one days, I was really lost. I had great problems with that. . . . Everything can blend into each other, the moments—because it's the same thing . . . it can all become one [duration of time] very easily.

Similarly, Carobeth Laird, who spent months in a nursing home, observes, "Because of the timeless monotony of institutional life, I have forgotten how long I was in The Ward. One week? Ten days? Two weeks?" (1979:53). She, too, alludes to unchanging time without meaning when she states, "Time dragged on in its peculiarly timeless way, which can certainly be understood only by those who have been confined in nursing homes or prisons" (1979:131). Yet a sense of unchanging time also develops whenever anyone experiences a lengthy immobilization from illness in a quasi-institutional setting.

As time slips away, existence and self also slip away. Hence, when conventional ways of marking and experiencing time dwindle, time, existence, and self disappear and may lose their meaning altogether. For Mark Reinertsen, keeping his transplant book did more than help him keep track of time; it also kept him grounded in the self he had possessed before. He explained, "It [keeping the transplant book] gave me a focus. And you really do need to keep a focus when you're in the hospital because you [the self] can float away so easily, float right out the window and on the floor; that's not very good. Yeah, and again I found that—it was the same thing with dialysis—having a focus in your life [that preserved his sense of self]."

Though most people echoed Mark Reinertsen's sentiments about losing self in a sea of unchanging time, not everyone wished to keep anchored to a past self. A few people reveled in the freedom that they found in loosening those anchors. A young woman who was influenced by Zen Buddhism elucidated: "My theory on time and space is that it's involved with ourselves as we experience them, and if you lose a sense of time and space you also lack a sense of self." She saw the self as a type of "bondage" that rivets one to worldly concerns. Being immersed in a stretched-out duration of illness had permitted her unexpected spiritual discovery and development.

Dragging and Drifting Time

When an individual is plunged into a serious episode, two main ways of experiencing time stand out: the dragging time of pain and suffering, and the drifting time of loss of consciousness. During the agony of pain, time lengthens. Moments expand and swell without end. No distractions—only pain, endless pain. As one woman said, "I'd thought I'd been lying there for hours, then I looked at the clock. Only twenty minutes had passed."

Suffering extends beyond the body; it also saps the spirit and fills the mind. Reminders of stigma, loss, or lack of control may also cause moments to stretch in length and to swell with meaning. When Harriet Binetti tried to answer her doctor's long-awaited call about her pain, her wheelchair got stuck on a cabinet. This incident compressed her pain, lack of control, and physical dependence into a protracted duration of time. She recounted, "I was here alone and . . . the phone was ringing; nobody heard me yell for help, but Sally [her attendant] had just gone to the store so she was back like right away, but not that quick. You know twenty minutes seems like twenty-two hours [then]."

Drifting time, in contrast, spreads out. Like a fan, drifting time unfolds and expands during a serious immersion in illness. This time is the elusive, slowed time when an immobile individual regains consciousness. Time drifts when action remains so limited. Yet drifting time also includes the amorphous, floating time when someone slips in and out of sleep or consciousness. Time elapses without awareness. Then, lengthy periods of clock-time collapse quickly into seemingly short durations. Here, the fan closes and durations fold without sequence. A woman whose condition had worsened described drifting time in this way: "It's a funny thing when I am that ill, time just moves; it drifts on. I don't remember much—I didn't think about dying, but I don't think about living either."

Immersion Time in Retrospect

Whether unchanging, dragging, or drifting, time seems different in retrospect than when experienced, depending upon whether immersion essentially ends or continues. If illness abates, then the prism of the present focuses views of the past (Maines, Sugrue, and Katovich 1983; Mead 1932). Thus, returning to "normal" pursuits results in changing images of the properties of one's past as well as one's present. The slow durations of a past episode of illness collapse and condense into a single event, which contrasts with present experience. For example, when I asked the young woman with colitis what the slow, unchanging time during her illness looked liked five years later, she quickly replied, "It seems like a wink."

As people collapse time in immersion, the length of their separation from their ordinary life seems to shorten. Whole periods of time can collapse into a forgotten void of experience, if health dramatically improves. In these circumstances, people distance their earlier immersion in illness from self, like a dream from which they feel dissociated. They return to their prior lives and selves as though never separated from them.

In contrast, when people believe that illness might reoccur, they may see a past immersion as a nightmare from which they must extricate themselves. A woman who had had cancer said, "I really don't like to go back into those memories; it was an extremely painful time." In her second interview, another woman said of the harrowing time when I first happened to interview her, "I don't want to think about how I was then; thinking about it might make it come back." These people disallow the content of the past to avoid repeating it in the future. They close that chapter of their lives and edit it from their biographies.

Memories of illness recede into the past when people can resume their earlier lives or involve themselves in new worlds with few reminders of the past illness. That way, they succeed in keeping their illness apart from self. Of course, having no further episodes of illness helps.

If someone does not improve, things look and feel quite differently. The slowing of time continues. Chronology blurs. After having had chronic fatigue syndrome for five years, Gregg Fisher explains, "The years since I've been ill are especially blurry. Part of the problem may lie in the fact that nothing terribly remarkable happens in my life anymore. Nothing changes, not even the symptoms of my illness. While healthy people's lives have memorable highs and lows, mine is static and stationary and lacking in memorable experiences" (1987:28).

After slipping into illness routines, people may find some comfort in their now familiar confinement. At least nothing worse happens. The future seems to spread out, but with the threat of danger and death. Subsequently, the self becomes wedded to the ritual of daily routines. These people hope that following their ritual will stave off further crises and death (Roth 1957). Yet, insulating oneself in routines can develop into a permanent accommodation to illness. If this occurs, the person probably cannot reinvent self or reconstruct a new life, even if his or her health improves substantially.

Variations in Immersion

A lengthy immersion in illness shapes daily life and affects how one experiences time. Conversely, ways of experiencing time dialectically affect the qualities of immersion in illness. The picture above of immersion and time has sharp outlines. What sources of variation soften or alter the picture of immersion and time? The picture may vary according to the person's: 1) type of illness, 2) kind of medications, 3) earlier time perspective, 4) life situation, and 5) goals.

The type of illness shapes the experience and way of relating to time. Clearly, trying to manage diabetes necessitates gaining a heightened awareness of timing the daily routines. But the effects of the illness may remain much more subtle. People with Sjögren's syndrome, for example, may have periods of confusion when they feel wholly out of synchrony with the world around them. For them, things happen too quickly, precisely when their bodies and minds function too slowly. Subsequently, they then may retreat into routines to protect themselves. Lupus patients usually must retreat because they cannot tolerate the sun. Sara Shaw covered her windows with black blankets when she was extremely ill. Thus, her sense of chronological time became further distorted as day and night merged together into an endless flow of illness.

Specific drugs alter time perspective and shape the experience of illness. Remaining oriented and maintaining a prior time perspective requires effort. Just after having another transplant, Mark Reinertsen mentioned, "I wasn't prepared for the psychological effects of the high dosages of cortisone, that it is a very spacey kind of drug; it makes it hard to concentrate on things." I asked, "What was time like for you?" He replied quickly, "It was totally disoriented and I would know more about that now and understand it, but I didn't expect that to that degree."

When people treasure having a finely tuned sense of clock-time, they actively resist relinquishing it despite being immersed in illness. They preserve ways of marking time from their past. For example, a housewife with multiple sclerosis charted and organized her days around her husband's work schedule and her children's schooling, as she had always done. She fit the routines of her substantial care around their schedules, rather than vice versa. A bookkeeper also tried to preserve his sense of clock-time. His days at home and at the convalescent hospital mirrored the order of his former workday. He timed and recorded his medications, food, and liquid in-take, as well as his sleep patterns and treatments in a log he kept as faithfully as he had kept the company books. Similarly, he scheduled visitors one at a time in an appointment book and refused to permit them to descend upon him unannounced.

Time perspective can also affect how readily someone becomes immersed in illness. Maintaining the chronology of earlier life helps to forestall such immersion. Conversely, inattention to chronology and clock-time hastens sliding into it and makes it easier to remain unaware of shifts in using time. Sara Shaw remarked, "I don't have any conception of what a year is, or two years is, or five years, or ten years. . . . I have never had a perception of time. . . . I know things that happened and I have a lot of memory, but I don't mark it; I don't have markers. . . . I never was good about remembering what day it was or things like that. And so I think I probably accepted it easier when I was sick."

A prior time structure similarly affects immersion. A tight time structure with multiple responsibilities forces awareness of—and most likely resentment about—being immersed in illness. A young woman felt frustrated about spending weeks in a darkened room because of lupus. She faced daily reminders of her inability to function. She could not go to work. She could not care for her toddler. She could not attend to the household tasks. She saw the debts rise because they had so little money.

She saw her daughter bond with her mother-in-law who cared for her. The continual disarray of the house and the steady diet of sandwiches testified, she felt, to her inability to function. With such tangible reminders of ties to a former time structure, one resists becoming lulled by the routines of illness.

Consequences of Immersion

Prolonged immersion in illness takes its toll—upon social relationships and self. If life winnows down to immediate bodily needs, a man or woman may turn inward to self and pose new questions for self.

Social Isolation

Being immersed in illness for lengthy periods isolates people. As illness recasts and redirects their lives, they lose common interests and no longer share pursuits with friends and associates from earlier days. And as they pull in to manage their illness, these others slip away from them. Immersion in illness erodes or entirely drowns most earlier friendships and casual relationships. In turn, losing contact fuels taking refuge in routines.

The resulting social isolation can be a natural sequel to illness. But the consequences of isolation are not entirely negative. One man discovered that it reduced distractions. Another man decided that many of his relationships had been superficial. Furthermore, isolation allows people to reduce pressures and to live at a tolerable pace. Before she became ill, Bonnie Presley had many friends and suitors. While immersed in illness, she observed, "My friends aren't close anymore. I don't know if it's me or what. . . . I still keep in touch, but I hardly ever see anybody. Since I moved here, I've become a hermit." I asked her, "How does that feel?" She replied, "It feels fine. I can pace myself. I try to keep all pressures away—no stress. I think that's important. Friends take time. It's unfortunate that you have to look at it like that."

Most people remain less sanguine about their shrinking social circles. When Mark Reinertsen was immobilized at home, he said, "I have an inner circle of close friends but I don't have that second circle of casual friends and acquaintances from which to replace them. There aren't many new people coming into my life."

Whether or not someone lives alone can crucially affect the degree of social isolation. Married people may have a family around them, although they often become isolated from friends, associates, and neighbors. Single people with relatives nearby also may have sustained contact with them. When the family consists of married children, however, visits may dwindle to brief checks and errands. An older woman who had been ill for over ten years reflected, "And the friends drift away; the relatives forget you, even your closest ones, when you are sick. Oh, everyone is all concerned when something happens and you are sick for a while, but if it lasts, if it is chronic, then they forget you and don't help you. Even my own children have never said, 'Mother, is there anything I can get you?' " (Charmaz 1973:35).

Generally, family provides the major buffer against social isolation. For this reason, single people without family nearby often find themselves quite isolated. Several single people created novel ways of developing or maintaining involvements and as a consequence received assistance and support when they needed it. Mark Reinertsen invited friends to potluck dinners at his house when he was too ill to leave. A middle-aged woman devised a schedule for several friends to make regular visits and phone checks. An elderly woman joined a telephone chain in which a volunteer called her at the same time every morning and she, in turn, called someone else each evening. Ostensibly, the service was designed to check on whether the person had suddenly deteriorated or died, but these elderly women used it to socialize. Their friendships blossomed as they listened to each other's tales about their families, health, and troubles.

Isolation accelerates in old age since many chronically ill elders' social horizons have already shrunk. Unless they possess substantial power, prestige, or property, they cannot bring the outside world into their homes. Even when ill people can bring outsiders in, try as they may, they seldom can keep them coming back beyond the specific task at hand. For example, an elderly man did not leave his house. When he decided to sell his huge library, he cultivated a relationship with the appraiser who also managed the sales. For a few months, the appraiser came every week or so to pay him and to visit. However, the visits dwindled and ended within a month after they finished their business.

Regular assistance, in contrast, offers better opportunities for social contact and for changing a formal relationship into an intimate one. Elderly people transform a home health aide or volunteer into a friend, or at least a welcome break in their routinized existence. An elderly man supplied the food that his home health aide fixed for both of them. After eating alone for many years, he enjoyed the companionship as they ate and watched television together. Bessie Thompkins elevated Stella, her home health aide, from a hired assistant to a friend to a family member. Because Stella had been divorced for a long time and had no children, Bessie included her in family holidays at her daughter's home and described Stella as a member of her family. Despite such creative efforts to reduce isolation, ill people's relationships typically dwindle and their worlds shrink.

Even superficial sociability can assume weighty symbolic significance to an isolated ill person. Such sociability affirms that the self remains, that illness has not claimed all of one's being. The significance of social contact lies in its *meaning*. Many ill people, especially elders, welcome social contact from whomever they can get it—the meals-on-wheels driver, the door-to-door missionary selling salvation, or the visiting nurse. Other people remain more aloof. Sadly, the infrequent phone calls of a son or daughter who never visits may mean more to an aged parent than solicitous daily care given by someone else (Calkins 1972). For them, time has definition and meaning only during the fleeting moments with a significant other.

Typically, social isolation translates directly into emotional isolation and loneliness (Lopata 1969). Loneliness intensifies when intimates identify the ill person as someone who has taken—or could take—over their lives. A daughter said of her seriously ill mother, "She's totally invasive, always been that way, and now that she is so sick, she not only has a reason for being invasive, she can really take over our lives." Hence, relatives decrease their involvement or they limit the "legitimate demands" that the ill person can make. Frequently, friends avoid being burdened with the ill person's loneliness. Further, friends and relatives tacitly define the ill person as someone whom they can treat in this circumscribed manner. Simultaneously, they may impart the double message of telling the person to ask for help. An elderly woman explained, "The attitude is, 'If I can do anything for you, just ask.' *But don't ask!* It is just an empty statement and they give you all these messages that you'd just better *not* ask. People say that to make themselves feel better, not you. And you had better not rely on them, or else you'll be awfully hurt, and maybe in a very bad pinch" (Charmaz 1973:36).

Certainly relatives' and friends' perceptions of the ill person affect the extent of their involvement. A fear of being overburdened might reflect a fear of illness and death. Also, strained interactions with the ill person can drive visitors away (Davis 1961). Without a social façade and superficial chitchat—that is, without safe discourse—being with the ill one can panic visitors. If someone refuses to talk about anything except the illness or will not talk at all, then just the most stalwart visitors keep coming.

Social isolation tends to be self-perpetuating. Isolation and immersion in a devastating illness foster the development of interactional styles that not only appear strange to others but serve to estrange them. For example, ill people can appeal to the sympathy or guilt of others through their "sad tales" (Goffman 1961a). Then, they try to trap family and friends into tighter bonds of intimacy or to entice new acquaintances into instant intimacy. In either case, this intimacy portends of extensive obligations. For a period, these others may attend to the ill persons simply because of the immediacy of their plight, or even because of guilt. But negative emotions grate, and guilt wears thin. Subsequently, an ill person may test others' loyalty and commitment precisely when they begin to ease themselves out of the relationship. Such testing intensifies the wish to drop the ill individual. Over time, ill people may come to believe that in order to reduce their isolation, they must force others to sense the pathos in their lives. Then should new acquaintances again happen to come these ill people's way, they repeat the scenario with renewed intensity and thus unwittingly perpetuate their own isolation.

Perhaps the most negative consequences of social isolation occur when people are poor and without access to social services. Poverty reinforces social isolation. In turn, poverty and social isolation trap people in a quagmire of immersion in illness (see Hopper 1981). Lacking both the social resources and the financial assets to help themselves, ill people can slip further and further into narrowed worlds and diminished lives.

Turning Inward

Increasing immersion in illness leads to becoming consumed by needs and feelings; people turn inward. Turning inward to self ranges from explicit, direct, and immediate focusing on the ill self to broader self-concerns that a person relates to illness. In the former, illness threatens to overtake or to overwhelm the individual—now. By the time he was thirty-seven, Mark Reinertsen's numerous acute illnesses, setbacks, and iatrogenic conditions had taken their toll. He disclosed, "I see myself as being on the edge. I feel fragile now. It's something that's cropped up in the last year. I feel older. I feel like an aged person. My body, whole body, creaks; it hurts like arthritis."

I said, "Tell me what being on the edge means to you." He reflected, "It's that feeling of not being in control; that's being on the edge. That's the hardest part—not that I am so active in my life. I don't work or go to school or anything. But just being able to get out and take a walk. . . . Not being able to make it across a full parking lot. Feeling that I couldn't make it is real scary."

"Being on the edge" for Mark also signaled his awareness of death, a death beyond his control. He said, "That fear has been getting stronger. I've noticed it. I've tried not to let it rule my life—the fear that I won't be in control, can't function. I don't know where it will end but at a certain point, I may decide not to stay around. I try not to let it worry me but. . . ."

When people turn inward, they retreat into self. A middle-aged man looked back at the onset of his illness twenty-three years before:

> I just got freaked out. I remember that I got—I don't know how to put it—I got sort of parsimonious, not really with money but with *myself*. It was like I had to stay here more [indicates close to his body], back here. That going out there [indicates away from his body] and not noticing what I was doing or how much I was laying out had nearly somehow been the undoing of me and now I had to consolidate and play my cards close to my chest and become circumspect.

Ill people turn inward to self primarily during crises, routine immersions, or whenever they lose hope. Doing so can point to a crisis of meaning. The man above recalled:

> I withdrew a lot. I got very afraid. I became very circumspect as I had not been before. Now in part, this was because I wasn't getting drunk anymore, I suppose. But it was just like—you know—I realized that I didn't lead a charmed life and disaster could strike me as anyone else, which had been an idea before that I had entertained but it is not the same as when you see that it is true.

As self-consciousness grows, ill people's awareness of others' needs often shrinks, even if they had been quite considerate earlier.[6] An older man told me, "My wife thinks I've become too demanding and expect too much help from her." Then, too, any prior tendency for self-involvement overpowers other concerns and fills the crevices of conversations.

A recurrence or spiraling complications may so involve ill people that they do not realize how immersed in illness they have become and how it has caused them to turn inward. During a visit from a close friend, Mark Reinertsen noted:

I realized I wasn't talking about anything *but* my medical problems. In one way it was OK because that's what was going on
anyway and so it is reasonable to share that with your friends
and on the other side, like for lately that's all they've been hearing and for me it sounds like all I've been saying. Then it's time
to stop and ask, "what is going on?" It seemed like that [illness]
was pretty much dominating my life.

Turning inward usually intensifies as someone moves closer
to death. Although many people cannot state their thoughts
and feelings directly, their faces and gestures dramatize their
concerns. A woman reported that her husband with emphysema coughed and moaned noticeably more and talked less
throughout a visitor's stay than he did otherwise. A man with
heart disease became distracted, depressed, and withdrawn,
his eyes mirrors of fear.

Identity Questioning

Identity questioning often results from immersion in illness.
Social isolation also can prompt identity questioning. Ill people
wonder where illness will take them and ask who they can be
during their odyssey—for self and for others. At this point,
illness serves as both foundation and focal point of their experience. Ill people ask:

Who will I be?
How will this condition affect my future?
How can I continue to be myself while having relentless
   illness?
What will being dependent do to me?

Thus, identity questioning means: 1) acknowledging the
identifications of self in the present, 2) comparing past identity
with that of the present, and 3) wondering what identity one
will have in the future. Hence, identity questioning involves
wondering if the present identity founded in illness will
become permanent and override other sources of identity.

Identity questioning can also include asking what was learned about self through illness and how to use it, should a return to a former life become possible.

Identity questioning can lead to feelings of being horrified and overwhelmed by one's body. To illustrate, a woman who experienced progressive deterioration said, "I couldn't believe it was me. Is this what I can expect?" In this case, the person learns that a past self may not be regained.

Dependency spurs identity questioning. The threat of permanent dependency strips away earlier self-definitions based upon independence. When facing another round of chemotherapy, one woman with cancer recalled her first immersion in illness. She said, "I was totally physically dependent on Norma [her lover] and I didn't like it. I didn't like it. That was worse than the treatment. I think I can face anything again but that feeling of total dependency. You lose yourself."

Many of the positive identifications of the past are swept or ripped away by illness. Without them, ill people become open to accepting the identifications imposed by others and may even seek them. As caregivers and medical functionaries gain control over ill people's experience, they may also control the defining images of ill people's selves. Yet these images may seem inconsistent with a past self. If that happens, then identity questioning develops.

Sometimes practitioners impose images of a discredited self widely divergent from an ill person's earlier self-concept (Goffman 1963). As the foundation of that earlier self crumbles, these images become real. A young woman described the discrediting evaluation she experienced in a medical clinic:

> You are raked across the coals and torn apart bit by bit until you are no longer the person you thought you were. It seems odd to me that if a person has a conscience at all, they feel bad enough about not working, or pursuing their studies to establish their independence, and then to be dependent on others when you used to be independent without being torn apart . . . whether you could do anything, no matter how conscientious—it all doesn't matter; they are clawing you apart. It is a shattering experience, especially if it is repeated. (Charmaz 1973:41)

This woman had already been shattered by illness and, therefore, looked to her physicians for some sign of hope for a more promising future. She said, "What else can you do [but let others define you] if you don't know who you are by then? . . . If your previous definition, or basis, or whatever, has been knocked all to smithereens, you are left with their definition—it's all you have" (Charmaz 1973:45).

Identity questioning also arises from having time to reflect, uninterrupted by the trivia of daily life. Here, identity questioning brings different lessons. Ill people gain a sense of resolution and self-awareness, despite the identities cast upon them. Bonnie Presley remarked:

> I dealt with a lot last year when I was sick because I think I had the time to do it. I had nothing else to do. You know, I wasn't working; I was in bed a lot. And what do you do if you're in bed a lot if you don't take drugs? I couldn't read. I couldn't concentrate. Yeah. So I just—my mind was just always thinking. I guess I worked out a lot of things.
> . . . What else did I work out? I guess overall would be self-acceptance. And I don't care if I'm married or not anymore. That I don't care if I have a man or not. That I've learned to accept that I can't push myself into being one thing, which I wanted to be. I'm a lot of things.

Losing the regularity of clock-time can allow for greater depth of thought. Sara Shaw welcomed the loss of clock-time: "Any kind of real thought, if you have to be interrupted every fifteen minutes, you're going to lose that [thought] anyway, and so in your life, how are you going to make—how are you going to do any real thinking on what you are and what your life is and things, if you have all these things, these markers, and these days and nights going on? [Laughs.] So I think it was—I don't think I fought that at all."

This immersion in illness then sparks an internal dialogue with self about self. Through the dialogue, people came to reject the negative images of self that earlier they had accepted. Instead, those images impelled them to discover and to define themselves. Under these conditions, identity questioning gives rise to a more resolute, immutable self, less swayed by social forces. For one woman, immersion in illness brought both a freeing of the spirit and a burdening of the self. She said:

> To me it's [immersion in illness] sort of moving toward spiritual states where you do lose a sense of self and time as a release. I mean self is a kind of bondage in a way—so it's wonderful—you move toward heaven—to not have that burden. But the other thing, of course, is that we are here. I exist as Jane so Jane comes back and wants to exist. So that's the hellish side. The thing is that you're kind of lost outside of time. . . . You can't get a grip on things. That was part of the helpless side of being sick is that time—you do feel that time is passing by in terms of being a human being and identity and something—we all feel like we have something to do. You feel like you're drifting; things aren't getting done; you're older.

P-A-R-T
II

Problems in Everyday Life

In Part I, I showed how people's experience of time changes when they have chronic illnesses. What ill people need to do in a day affects their experience of time. The day shortens when chronic illness imposes a set of chores and needs upon an already hectic schedule. The day lengthens when ill people's activities shrink to waiting to get well or to improve. In Part II, I turn to practical problems of living with chronic illness.

Chapter 5 considers the problems that ill people face in talking about their conditions. They find that how and when to tell other people pose perturbing problems—repeatedly. The fact of illness can take on enormous significance for images and definitions of self. A shocking diagnosis, an invisible impairment, a growing disability, a terminal prognosis can make telling and talking frightful and painful. Practical problems in telling and talking mirror the meanings of illness for the emerging self. When the meanings are heavy ones, people often agonize over telling others about their illnesses. I emphasize this type of telling since so many of my respondents dwelled upon it.

Yet meanings change if illness recedes into the background of life. Hence, someone may talk openly about a diagnosis at first, selectively, if diminished by other people's judgments, and scarcely at all, if much time passes between episodes.

In Chapter 6, I discuss living with chronic illness and expand upon the problems in reordering time that occur when illness becomes intrusive. In Chapter 3, I described what an intrusive illness means. In Chapter 6, I look at how people live with an intrusive illness. All the logistical problems of planning, organizing, pacing, and juggling necessitated by a chronic illness blend with everyday life, often in taken-for-granted ways. Throughout the chapter, I focus on how people adapt themselves and their days and, sometimes, invent ways to handle their lives. Certainly, major ways of adapting include narrowing one's *pursuits, eliminating tasks, and staying home. These adaptations may occur so gradually or coincide so exactly with other life changes, such as retirement, that people may remain unaware of the effects of illness.*

In contrast, immediate responsibilities like raising children and getting to work often prompt people to give explicit scrutiny to planning shortcuts and timesavers. Because regimens blend with everyday life, I treat them as part of the daily work with which ill people concern themselves. Whether people invent strategies to help them remain active or adapt by slowing down, daily living with chronic illness provides important lessons about ill people's developing selves.

5

Disclosing Illness

I think that emotionally I would feel like if I got sick again that the same stuff would happen again in terms of that I would be real alone, and that I would have to deal with everything alone, that I couldn't tell anyone that I was sick and that I wouldn't be able to take care of myself, but that I wouldn't be able to ask for help. And to be in that is a real double bind, you know?

Sara Shaw became ill sixteen years ago. After several years of having her symptoms discounted, she received a diagnosis of lupus erythematosus, which was changed to mixed collagen disease five years ago. She made the above statement nine years ago. Two years after that interview, she said, "If I were to start going with somebody pretty heavily, how would I tell them about having been sick, the possibility that I could be sick again—that scares me to death." I asked, "So it's not something that comes up in your friendships?" She said:

> Yeah, actually everyone that I've talked to or been real close to that I'm friends with, I've told that I *was* sick. I don't tend to say that I am sick now. I don't tend to say it in terms of the present tense, or in terms of an ongoing, a chronic, illness. . . . But I also wonder if anyone would understand if I were to get involved with somebody to the point of marriage, the point of sharing lives. I have very little balance on that question.

Three years later, Sara disclosed, "I don't think I do trust anybody in terms of letting them know about having been sick, even though I'm not sick now. That's something like that is kind of secret." Subsequently, two years later, seven years after her first statement above, she remarked:

107

It's [her illness and near-death experience] like a prestige thing now, I mean that I've gone through a near-death experience at ALU [the university where she worked] is like, I mean I'm one level higher, you know, for that. . . . That comes out quickly, you know, in whatever way it comes out. That started [for her] with FPI [a psychological institute specializing in intensive workshops using simulated families to work on family-of-origin issues]. . . . I was able to bring that out and say I had a lot of fears . . . around having—being intimate and letting people know, you know, that I had had, that I get sick sometimes and because I talked to them about everything, the people that I'm close to in that family. . . . I never thought I could say stuff like that because then I thought that they would need, they would feel that they would need to change me, or heal me, or fix me. And we don't have to do that to each other, we're just sharing our lives, that's it, you know. So that's real new. Yeah, but I do that now. I'm not seeing anybody romantically, so I haven't had to deal with that. Uhm, but I think I would tell because what's happened is I'm not willing enough to abandon myself to where I wouldn't bring that up. I would want someone to know now.

To tell or not to tell? How much to tell? Risk disclosure but face rejection? Sara Shaw pondered over these questions for years. When she first became ill, the young man with whom she lived left three days before her exploratory surgery. Later, when her doctor told her that she would need care, she found that she had no one on whom she could rely. Not surprisingly, she grew secretive about her past illness and any present symptoms. Disclosing illness meant heavy risks.

For Sara Shaw, like others, disclosing illness meant revealing her feelings and vulnerabilities. Disclosing is a form of telling in which someone reveals self. When one discloses illness, facts and feelings about it touch one's self-concept and self-esteem (Jourard 1971; Zerubavel 1982). Still, an individual's stance toward disclosure may change with time, as Sara's did, as experiences change and as new perspectives are gained.

How do chronically ill people handle telling others about their illnesses? What does disclosure and avoiding disclosure mean to them?[1] When do they disclose? How do they manage their emotions about disclosing? What concerns do ill people have about others' responses to their disclosures?

Dilemmas of Disclosing Illness

Chronically ill people wonder what they *should* tell and what they *need* to tell others about their illnesses. Kathleen Lewis, who has lupus erythematosus, begins her book, " 'How are you?' can perhaps become the most difficult question a chronically ill person needs to learn to answer" (1985:3). Telling anything about illness can mean revealing potentially discrediting information about self (Schneider and Conrad 1980; 1983). Telling often means exposing hidden feelings. Telling sometimes means straining relationships. Telling can also mean risking loss of control and autonomy (Cozby 1973). Hence, some men and women will not tell family, friends, and associates that they have a chronic illness, and many others avoid updating people about their conditions. Other ill people take the risk or feel compelled to apprise select individuals about their situations.

Telling does not end. Physicians can impart bad news and depart (Clark and La Beff 1982; Glaser 1966; Glaser and Strauss 1965; Sudnow 1967; Taylor 1988). Unlike physicians, chronically ill people must tell and retell their news to many people and frequently do so at each step along the path that their illness takes. Moreover, they must live with the telling.

Perhaps most fundamentally, young and middle-aged adults risk losing acceptance by telling; older adults risk losing autonomy. Young and middle-aged adults can find themselves ignored, rejected, and stigmatized when they disclose their illnesses (Goffman 1963; Hopper 1981; Schneider and Conrad 1983). Not only must they handle their feelings about telling, but also they must handle their feelings about another's response to being told. Lovers, spouses, friends, and jobs may vanish from their lives. Of course, older adults experience these responses, too, but many older adults, particularly single elderly women, already have only a frail hold on their autonomy. Adult children or service providers, concerned about the safety of these elderly people or the quality of their housekeeping, may see their illness as a reason to grasp more control over them. For these older adults, telling means losing control over their homes, their mobility, their money, their decisions—in short, their lives. Meanwhile, they also must handle losing their health.

Thus, the dilemmas of disclosing turn on control—control of identity, control over information, control over emotional response, and control over one's life. Hence, avoiding disclosure entirely, maintaining distance, metering disclosures, censoring information, and pacing disclosures all become ways of preserving control.

Avoiding Disclosure

Given the potential costs, avoiding disclosure can be a natural response to illness. Avoiding disclosure takes a different twist than concealing illness. When people avoid disclosure, they try to circumvent or minimize others' attending to their health status. Concealing illness often takes an enormous amount of commitment, planning, and work. When people conceal illness, they shroud it in secrecy. Avoiding disclosure can be easier and may reflect a spontaneous decision during the course of a conversation. By avoiding disclosure, people try to keep their illness understated in a relationship, or in their lives, more generally. Certainly an underlying reason for either concealing illness or for avoiding disclosure turns on whether someone grants illness any reality at all, and, if so, what kind of reality.

Both concealing illness and avoiding disclosure distance illness from the self and avoid stigma. Yet a serious exacerbation can puncture a long-maintained secrecy. As her disability progressed, Tina Reidel tried to hide it in public and, thus, attempted to avoid stigma. During a recent interview, she described the embarrassment she had felt that morning when she could hardly walk through a department store:

> When I got up, after having my makeup done, I felt like I could hardly walk and I kept thinking, "I hope nobody notices, you

know, that I'm really this way, that I can hardly walk." . . . It's like I think that other people could perceive the way I perceive myself, but they can't. So it's like I try to keep it hidden. . . . I think it's real embarrassing. You know, like say if someone can see that I can hardly walk or something, I'm all stooped over or you know, I catch a glimpse of myself in ah, like a window, it's very shocking sometimes what I see.

I asked, "In which way?" She said:

Well, I can see that, other people can see is that, you know, my leg, I can hardly walk on it. And I feel like somehow I'm not a whole person and . . . people can look at it and feel sympathetic, but they can look at you and see you as being less than whole, you know. . . . And ah, it's frightening, I guess. . . . This idea of getting foot surgery and it's really scary because I don't think I'd be able to walk for about three months; I'd have to wear those bunny boots [removable casts]. And just the idea of like trying to go out in the world and it being like more apparent, that's the scariest part. It's not so much the pain I'd go through or anything, it's just that they'd *know*. It's like I'd be—you know, people could *see*.

A visible disability does not permit choice about whom to tell, when to tell, or how to tell. Under these conditions, information about self once held private becomes public knowledge and floods *self* as well as potentially flooding interaction. At that point, ill people often feel forced to face their feelings and values about disability.

Until disability becomes a visible and continuing fact, someone who avoids disclosure can more readily treat illness as a temporary interruption, rather than as a chronic condition. The possibility of effective medical procedures in the future can further this stance. For example, a kidney dialysis patient looked well, functioned quite well at work, and believed that he was in much better shape than other patients on the dialysis unit. Since he did not want to be identified as ill or disabled, he told no one beyond his family about his illness. He said, "I'm not really ill at all from this thing. And I'm perfectly able to keep working. It takes a little time to be on the machine, but I just schedule around it. It's really a very minor part of my life. And who knows? A transplant might become available and then this [dialysis] will be over."

Further, avoiding disclosure limits the reality of illness to self and for others. Lara Cobert recalled her first episode: "I remember not talking a lot about it, not telling a lot of people. Talking about it would make it real and I didn't want to think of it as permanent." Thus, avoiding disclosure allows claiming other identities than illness. To the extent that concealing illness and avoiding disclosure work, these strategies limit stigma and support preferred self-images.

Perhaps more commonly, ill people refuse to grant illness legitimacy to shape their lives and self-concepts. They do not wish to exploit their illness to their advantage. Bonnie Presley toyed with telling her accounting teacher that her illness had prevented her from completing an assignment. She said, "It's almost like you'd be using it, do you know what I mean? It sort of feels like that. You know about—with teachers—you hear about all these teachers and they say this guy said this and this girl said this and 'I have so many people lose their grandmothers,' and, you know, all these excuses for not doing their work. But everybody else has reasons too why they can't get it done, so I'm no different."

People with invisible illnesses often refused to grant legitimacy to the special needs that their illnesses engendered, and therefore, they chose not to disclose. Occasionally, they deferred to someone else's physical needs. For example, when the elevator stopped running just before my seminar, a student who used a wheelchair phoned to request that the class meet on the lawn. The class members agreed but several weeks later, a student who had multiple sclerosis told me, "I should have never gone out with the class; it was just too hot for me that day and I can't take the heat, but at the time, I thought Connie's needs were greater than mine. So I didn't say anything."

Potential Losses and Risks

In addition to the ultimate risks of losing acceptance and autonomy, ill people face immediate interactional risks: 1) being rejected and stigmatized for disclosing and for having an illness (cf. Ponse 1976), 2) being unable to handle others' responses, and 3) losing control over their emotions.

When people believe that they risk losing—or assuredly will lose—status or self-esteem, they avoid disclosing illness. Lin Bell would not tell her co-workers when she had angina attacks. Instead, she tried to hide when she took her nitroglyercine so that her temporary distress would remain unnoticed. However, her tactics did not always work. She said:

> Somebody saw me and you know how word gets around. I was hiding behind a cage, kind of bent over, taking [the pill]—well she went running to the supervisor and he sent somebody else over to see how I was doing—I was just having an angina attack. No worse than what I had before the heart attack. Now they're scared to death I'm going to have one there. And I don't want them to think that I can't keep up, 'cause they don't have to give me a light duty assignment. There's a lot of pressures in this world.
>
> The people who'll support me are fine—it's—it's the ones who think they're being my friend by running and saying, you know, "Watch Lin, she'll go lay down or something." If I do—if they do that too often, the . . . [management] is going to say, "Hey, let's get her out of here. Why pay $13.00 an hour to somebody who can't keep up?"

Most men and women want to be known for attributes other than illness. Therefore, they will conceal illness or avoid disclosures when they see that illness could cloud other people's images and judgments of them. They will not take the risk. Because photojournalist Roger Ressmeyer would not allow his diabetes to flood his identity, he decided not to disclose it at work. During one incident, he risked possible residual brain damage or even death from insulin shock rather than request minimal help—and thereby disclose his illness. He writes:

> I had forgotten to bring some food along. I napped intermittently, vaguely more aware that the insulin injection I had taken earlier that morning was reaching its peak and my need for food was becoming critical. But I was too tired and embarrassed to mention my rapidly worsening condition to the well-known

news photographer next to me, or to the driver or to anyone who might have had the apple or candy that would have saved me.

When I awoke, as from a dream, I was horrified to discover that I was standing on the street in front of a deli in Cocoa Beach with a half-empty bottle of orange juice in my hand. My head was throbbing and my body was shuddering. Hours had obviously passed, since the printed image of the shuttle launch stared at me from a newspaper rack. I had no recall of walking to the deli, or the missing hours. Many diabetics have accidents under exactly the same conditions but some angel must have been watching me. (1983:8)

Knotty problems, shaky relationships, and harsh judgments make disclosing a dilemma. Subsequently, people avoid disclosing for months, or even years. To an older woman, her husband's alcoholism and consequent chronic illnesses seemed much more pressing than her own illness and growing disability. Though she had known for five years that she had lupus erythematosus, she had not told her husband about it. Tenuous or hostile relations can also increase an individual's proclivity not to tell. For example, a middle-aged man with cancer faced an uncertain future. Three years earlier, he had divorced his wife after a hostile separation and nasty legal battle. Although he had severed contact with her and their daughter, he continued to feel unrelenting rage toward his ex-wife whom, he believed, had poisoned their daughter against him. He vowed that the first news either of them would have about his illness would be in his obituary.

Fear of being thought of as a complainer or whiner dissuades people from discussing their illnesses. Christine Danforth said:

If you have lupus, I mean one day it's my liver; one day it's my joints; one day it's my head, and it's like people really think you're a hypochondriac if you keep complaining about different ailments. . . . It's like you don't want to say anything because people are going to start thinking, you know, "God, don't go near her, all she is—is complaining about this." And I think that's why I never say anything because I feel like everything I have is related one way or another to the lupus but most of the people don't know I have lupus, and even those that do are not going to believe that ten different ailments are the same thing. And I don't want anybody saying, you know, [that] they don't want to come around me because I complain.

A tendency to avoid disclosure intensifies when ill people had not talked about previous illnesses or feelings. Christine Danforth's father had died a painful death from cancer, but no one in the family had ever discussed his pain and suffering. Similar patterns repeat themselves. Christine believed that her mother knew her diagnosis but not what it meant. Not only did Christine resist revealing her discomfort, but also, when she did disclose, others did not believe her. She said, "My friends would call and say 'Let's go here or let's go there,' and I'd say, 'I can't; I just can't walk,' and they'd say, 'Pulling another Elise [her sister who as a child used her back injury as an excuse to get out of chores], huh?' So I never, ever would say that I hurt when they called. Ever."

Once ill people have proof that others will use their disclosures against them, they guard against disclosing. Even people who had earlier revealed their feelings, as well as their conditions, become circumspect and guarded after discovering that someone used their disclosures against them. Patricia Kennedy recalled that for a lengthy period, "I became very, very careful." Like many other ill people, she learned to answer questions about how she was feeling by saying, "I'm fine."

Having a condition that everyone "knows" about raises special risks of disclosing. These conditions elicit probing questions about health habits and regimen, which, in turn, can escalate into continuing criticism. Though irritating enough to have one's private behavior relegated to public discourse and evaluation, the criticism can sting already open wounds. And when this happens, the judgments stick. Such criticism reflects an objectified version of similar silent inner dialogues ill people have long had in which they berate themselves about their difficulties or failures in following their regimens. Lin Bell remarked:

I think the not telling is that I smoke. . . . I am so guilty for that. And yet I'm not willing to quit. And when you tell somebody you smoke and you have heart disease, a little computer in their head goes, "Hey, this person is self-destructive," and I'm tired of hearing that, 'cause I'm not. I know that I'm smoking, Kathy; I know that it doesn't help me. But I am not self-destructive. I don't have a death wish at all.

Risking disclosure extends into whether to claim having special needs, or to acknowledge hardships, long after everyone knows the diagnosis. Maureen Murphy's employers had forced her to take a disability leave for a year because of her diagnosis of multiple sclerosis. When she returned to work, they switched her to a less physically demanding job in another department with much less pay. After not working for a year, she felt grateful to have a job at all and therefore concealed any indication that the work was too strenuous for her. She recalled, "When I first started [working] there, I was doing filing and that got me tired, but I remember, you know, 'cause they didn't know what—where I would fit in, and so they decided to let me file for a little. And I didn't dare say a thing about being tired because I thought, 'Oh, God, they'll bounce me out of here,' you know. And, oh, that first day I was ready to drop."

Similar issues arise in relationships. For example, his respiratory therapist observed that keeping pace with his much healthier wife wore out a sixty-eight-year-old man with emphysema and heart disease. But he wouldn't tell his wife that he needed to slow down because he felt so guilty about draining their finances for his care. He wanted, at least, to help her with daily chores. He risked more rapid deterioration to gain a more favorable image in her eyes. For single ill people, the mere thought of repeatedly explaining their inability to maintain a new friend's pace can stifle romantic involvement.

Conceptions of illness as private lead to avoiding disclosure. For many people, facts and feelings about illness rank with sex and finances for deserving privacy. Maintaining this privacy becomes part of a creditable self. Bonnie Presley remarked, "I'd like to feel better before I have a relationship. I guess maybe I'm not willing to share it." I asked, "Share it?" She said:

Share when I don't feel good—share things like that. I'm not willing—I mean I don't tell my daughter very often—I *don't* tell her. . . . I know people who call and tell me real personal things and I just think, "God, this person doesn't even know me and you're telling me that?" I can't do that.

It's [feeling ill]; it's private; it's mine. In a relationship, you'd have to share. If somebody doesn't feel good and they don't want to talk about it, then living alone seems like the answer. You don't have to explain.

Should family, friends, and acquaintances think that the person's illness, treatments, or symptoms are stigmatizing, they may demand that he or she keep quiet about them. Thus, avoiding disclosure naturally follows. Ill people, like this woman who had a bowel dysfunction, find "that I can talk about this disease but that I can't find anyone to listen." Although she spoke freely about her pain and sudden diarrhea to immediate co-workers, they cut her off. She needed support and care from her lover, but he could not tolerate the dirt and disorder her condition caused and therefore he either ignored or castigated her. As Mitteness (1987) points out, bodily control is a prerequisite to competent adult status. Thus, the lack of such control goes beyond forcing disclosure; it threatens to elicit judgments of inadequacy and incompetence. To the extent that others impose their judgments and that ill people share them, they will avoid both disclosures and situations in which their symptoms might become apparent (Conrad 1987; Mitteness 1987; and Reif 1975).

Even without having symptoms that undermine bodily functions, ill people often fear negative responses, revealed through direct statements, gestures, and tone. Usually after their first serious episode, ill people will tell everyone all the details about their illness, hospitalization, and doctor's advice. Although initially interested, other people soon weary of these conversations and begin to treat the ill person as diminished, a malingerer, or an object of fleeting pity. Occasionally, ill people's friends and acquaintances told them that they looked "better" but their tone and expression belied their statements. Not surprisingly then, ill people prop themselves up for social occasions with the help of their closest intimates. They try to present a public face preserved from the past, only to collapse when they return home (Bury 1982). While still convalescing, an older man with heart disease attended the office Christmas party. He attempted to look as vigorous as possible. He rested for long hours before, dressed nattily, rehearsed a ready repetoire of jokes and quips, and minimized any overexertion in getting there. Afterwards, he spent three days recovering from the event. By preserving a public face, these people avoid or mini- mize others' negative judgments that link their state of health with their being. Preserving an earlier public face also protects a current self-conception. To the extent that ill people preserve that public face, they can more easily maintain the same feelings about self.

By modifying certain disclosures, metering some disclosures, and censoring still others, an individual can provide continuity with a past self or protect a now fragile or vulnerable self. After a turbulent first marriage that ended with her husband's death, a young widow looked forward to a happy second marriage. She asked her fiance if he could be happy with someone who could not play tennis with him. She had a minor, but visible, disability and high fatigue. Though her doctor had diagnosed her as having multiple sclerosis, she vascillated between not accepting the diagnosis and doubting it. To her, doubting the accuracy of the diagnosis justified not telling her fiance about it. She said, " 'cause I do wonder about this [having MS], you know. I think the hardest thing is for me not knowing really whether I have it or not, so I can't see whether I should, you know, make things—jeapardize things by saying that." By avoiding this disclosure, she maintained continuity with a pre- ferred self but risked later recriminations and feeling guilty about deception.

Interaction with others may lead an ill person to censor disclo- sure. For example, after a woman had snubbed Tina Reidel, she then censored her disclosures. She recalled, "When she next asked how my arthritis was, I said really quickly, '*Don't ask.*' " She reflected:

> Some people I feel I can bring in. Other people I have to keep out. . . . When they see me, it's as if they are thinking all these other thoughts—like, "should I go up to her?" or "what's she

thinking?" They're thinking about me—I can pick it up. But they're not spontaneous. They don't just go, "Oh, hi, Tina," or "Good to see you." Like that girl who knew me; I thought it was very awkward for her to stand in front of me and talk to the other person and not acknowledge me. So what it equates in my mind is: Why should I bare my vulnerability to this person? They don't even care.

Forms of Telling

Telling means relating thoughts, actions, or feelings with sufficient clarity to be understandable. Telling usually includes announcing and recounting professionals' accounts of one's illness and prognosis. Because disclosing represents a subjective form of telling, the person's experiencing, feeling self is brought into the foreground. Private views of self and personal dilemmas seldom made public in middle-class American life may emerge.

I discovered two ways of disclosing: protective disclosing and spontaneous disclosing. Protective disclosing is designed to control how, what, when, and who people tell about their illness. They intend to protect others and themselves from shock, anger, and fear about their illness and its future implications. In addition, protective disclosing helps to reduce another's anger or frustration about his or her unfulfilled expectations of the ill person. When effective, protective disclosing controls the form and timing of information, softens its potential harshness, and buffers everyone's emotions about it. Since protective disclosing typically necessitates planning, I describe it separately.

Spontaneous disclosing includes full expression of raw feelings, open exposure of self, and minimal or no control over how, when, where, what, and whom to tell (Schneider and Conrad 1983).[2] People spontaneously disclose when they receive startlingly bad news or perceive dramatic changes. Their view of self does not reflect the self mirrored by illness. Soon after relocating to another area, Joanne Dhakzak received a diagnosis of lymphoma. She called two old friends, "We're good friends but we don't keep in that close contact. I remember calling them and it was like I was trying to acknowledge and accept the fact that I did have this. . . . It was like I *had* to tell somebody and I had to have somebody tell me it was going to be okay."

Occasionally, spontaneous disclosing accompanies good news, such as when someone learns that he or she will receive a kidney transplant. At that point, friends and acquaintances might learn more about the individual's feelings about having renal failure than they had during the entire length of the illness.

More commonly, people with life-threatening illnesses pour out their concerns and feelings when they first realize what their diagnoses might mean, if they can talk about their illness at all. When they do talk about it, their fear, sorrow, rage, or self-pity may flood the interaction. Several people echoed this remark: "I was babbling about it [her illness]." Later, they usually feel mortified for having dealt with the news in that way, at that time, or to that person.

Illness, uncertain decline, and death can consume an ill person's thoughts entirely. Subsequently, any hint or comment reminding the person of illness calls forth more uncontrolled revelations. Joanne Dhakzak recalled, "For the first couple of years, it seemed like I'd tell everybody; it would just happen to come up in a conversation and I always managed to get it in—I mean if it would work in logically, I'd manage to get it in. Not with strangers, but the people at work."

Feelings about illness swell and resurface. Reconciling these feelings becomes difficult when an ill person also views them as no longer appropriate. After having had no recurrence for five years, Joanne Dhakzak wanted to see herself as recovered. Yet she felt that she dwelled too much on her illness. She viewed her spontaneous disclosures as testimony to her unresolved feelings about her illness and to her fear of recurrence: "I'd like to be able to be in a group conversation and somebody mentions cancer, have me think to myself, 'yeah,' and then go on to something else instead of going, 'Me too!' and on and on and on. I want to be able to put it into proper perspective, or what I feel is proper perspective, and *pull* it out when I want to, but not have it just always *spring* out."

Spontaneous disclosing turns into self-exposure as an ill individual reveals strong feelings and raises sticky questions about self, significant others, and situation. For example, a forty-seven-year-old woman with multiple sclerosis raged against her husband who had left her during her first debilitating episode three years before. She disclosed to anyone who would listen, "My husband walked out during the first year I had this. There I was lying in bed all the time and he up and leaves. He didn't even last the first year of this and that wasn't the worst of it either [her illness]—I wasn't even in a chair then. He hasn't sent me a cent; I haven't heard from him—not one word. Not even a card. Now what kind of a person would do that?"

When informing, in contrast, ill people assume an objective stance, almost as if their bodies and their situations remain separate from themselves. And, in fact, this objective stance reflects some people's experience of illness. To them, threatening complications lie in a distant future, if at all. They apprise others of their health status and impart "facts" to them. They neither view informing as risky, nor do they view themselves as discreditable for having an illness. Often, they wish to tell people how to minimize getting their illness, what having it is like, or how their lives resemble everyone else's. For example, Heather Robbins told everyone about having multiple sclerosis. She said offhandedly, "I'm a mother; I'm a wife; I'm a student; I also have MS." In a later interview, she said, "I try to educate people about MS, that it is not such a horrible disease."

Informing decreases emotional risks. Compared to disclosing, informing permits greater control over emotions, over others' responses, and over possible negative labels. For example, her friend recalled how Helen Bartlett informed her about having leukemia. The friend said, "Helen got very technical but there was no crack in her voice. That's Helen. She doesn't even give you a chance to think she's going to die" (Clark et al. 1985:69).

Through strategic announcing, ill people extend their control over the information, themselves, and another's response. They *organize* what they will tell, to whom they will tell it, and when they will do it. Strategic announcing can protect self, control interaction, and preserve power (Derlaga and Grzelak

1979; Goffman 1975; Schlenker 1980; Wilsnack 1980). Strategic announcing takes a stronger cast than informing. Frequently, people use these announcements to make declarations to wider, more public audiences. Therefore, they must study and shape ongoing interaction in order to be effective. For example, Mark Reinertsen learned that he probably would lose his kidney transplant. During a class discussion on quality of life, he introduced the dilemma of being tied to a dialysis machine. He announced, "Most of you don't know this, but I have a kidney transplant and it looks like I am about to lose it. I'm not sure that it's worth living if I have to go back on dialysis. And I'd really like some input on that."

Because control and power are the very attributes challenged, diminished, or lost when one is ill, strategic announcing can further attempts to maintain control and power. By making an effective strategic announcement, an individual controls and directs interaction, conflict, and outcome—and at the same time presents and protects self, or even creates an advantage over someone else.

Repeated strategic announcements, artfully placed, offer protection from the demands, expectations, and assumptions of others. Strategic announcements become necessary 1) when illness remains unacknowledged, ignored, or minimized by others, and 2) when illness requires someone to get help or to reduce previous obligations. Invisible illnesses can necessitate repeated strategic announcing to inform, enlighten, remind, and instruct others.

Invisible illnesses, intermittent illnesses, or minor disabilities can cause losses in strength, endurance, and function that only a practiced eye might see. Subsequently, friends, family, and co-workers discount the person's illness or fail to comprehend how it affects him or her, even when "informed." The sister of a woman with lupus erythematosus said, "We always thought she was just a complainer." Disappointment, strain, and confrontation follow. "Why aren't you carrying your share of the load?" "How come you don't just take the bus rather than expecting me to drop you at the door?" "How come it takes you so long to get dinner on the table? You've been here all day!"

Tina Reidel realized that her lover and his adult son, who

lived next door, neither understood, nor even acknowledged, her pain from rheumatoid arthritis. She strategically announced her pain to teach them how it affected her and to alter their perceptions of her actions. When walking past her lover's son without stopping to chat, she said, "I'm in a lot of pain today." She intended to explain her abruptness and to instruct him not to make demands on her. Because she felt that they hardly acknowledged her illness, she made multiple announcements about being interviewed for a research project on experiencing chronic illness. For her, being interviewed meant objective validation of her claims to having a serious chronic illness.

Strategic announcing can boost self-presentation or display self-importance. This happens when ill people announce significant events surrounding past or present episodes of illness. They retell these events to startle or to elicit concern from their audience (Zurcher 1982). Vera Mueller explained, "Who else at twenty-one years old had open heart surgery? It is one of those little things that sets me off and makes me different. It's great. I love it. 'Oh yeah, when I was 21, I had open heart surgery,' and people go, 'Uhh, you're kidding.' Yeah, it's wonderful. It's an ice-breaker at parties; it does great things."

Such an announcement rivets others' attention and concern and shapes the subsequent interaction and the emotional climate of the situation. The more dramatic the announcement, the more attention and feeling it elicits. The ill person gains sympathy, a sense of uniqueness, and sometimes—desired or not—pity.

Earlier crises can serve as identity badges to display when potentially useful and, especially, to teach others of one's hidden value: "they [doctors and hospital staff] did all this for little old me." Illness also provides gauges for measuring the quality of relationships. A hospitalization, for example, provides a gauge by which one can measure loyalty, devotion, and commitment. Obviously, who shows and who helps during a hospitalization are ready measures. When Lin Bell had her second angioplasty, her current date, Lotta, sat with her through the night. Lin said, "And she had to go to work the next day. I'll never forget that from her. I really appreciated that."

Strategic announcing, of course, is not limited to ill people.

Apparently, Lotta made her own announcement, which broke up the relationship, but provided Lin Bell's physicians with information. She recounted:

> So then Dr. Howard was saying, "And you've quit smoking," and "Oh, Dr. Martin's so proud of you," blah, blah, and I'm saying "Yes, yes." And Lotta's sitting there saying, "Lin, tell the truth, you have to tell these doctors the truth," and I was thinking, "Oh, God, I'd like to bat you right in the mouth." And so she takes little Dr. Howard outside the door and goes, "And she is smoking, doctor."

How staff responds to an ill person can also stand as a useful measure of their commitment. Lin Bell recalled Dr. Howard's response: "He just looked at me—he's cute—he just looked at me and said, 'Well, you know Dr. Martin and I are not going to quit treating you, because a lot of doctors would quit 'cause you're smoking.' "

Certainly, the "wrong" images of self can emerge when someone else does the announcing. To teach the proper meanings of self and illness effectively, one must also time strategic announcements well. By announcing either too early or too late, an ill person may lose a strategic advantage. A middle-aged man told his co-workers too early. They then scrutinized his work for signs of slipping and hinted that he could be a drain on them. By the time he actually needed their assistance several years later, they had solidified their position against giving help. Similarly, announcements lose their strategic effect when they come too late. Other people already see the results of illness and account for them in their dealings with the person. Worse yet, their spontaneous responses can proclaim a rapid decline. "What the hell happened to you?" "My God, how you've aged!" These exclamations beg for explanations. By this point, however, any announcement only eliminates rude questions, rather than providing strategic advantage.

Ill people make strategic announcements to control interaction and expectations. As Tina Reidel mentioned, "I can use it [illness] to put up as a block not to deal with someone I don't particularly care for. I do use it, but it's like the illness, to me, is more important, mine, you know, than the relationship with that person. I always think in my mind, 'Well, I don't care if I ever see them again.' "

Ill people can also use strategic announcements to coerce friends and family into doing something that they otherwise would not do. Enlisting a partner to disclose can strengthen the message. For example, with her homebound husband's approval, a woman called his son who was in arrears on a joint loan. She announced to the son, "The doctor said that all this stress he is having over the loan may kill him."

In this instance, as in others, strategic announcing can be used to elicit guilt and responsibility. This stepmother believed that her stepson ought to feel guilty about letting his father down and about "causing" yet more serious symptoms. She also wanted to nudge him to come through with the loan payment immediately. Sometimes an ill person tries to elicit guilt and responsibility for less tangible reasons, like having good health and not sharing his or her fate. By nurturing the seeds of guilt, an ill person might also be able to build a foundation for extracting later commitments for care. Using guilt effectively relies on shared definitions of the situation, the relationship, and the consequent "correct" behavior. Thus, from the start, an ill person must strategically reaffirm his or her definitions.

Strategic announcements to elicit guilt can become a pattern. A fear of decline and death spurs turning each episode into a "crisis," which therefore justifies receiving help. When no help is readily forthcoming, ill people may increase their strategic announcements and appeals to guilt. Whether real or contrived, repeated crises lead all but the most committed, or the most manipulated, family members and friends to abandon these ill people unless death is certain. Those who abandon them decline the appeals to guilt and refuse to be taught.

How, when, and to whom ill people make strategic announcements can serve as symbolic statements of others' relative position, prestige, and priority. The meaning of these statements intensifies when an ill individual holds considerable power within a family or group. Whether young or middle-aged, children, particularly, note their relative status when a parent makes announcements.

Strategic announcing reflects motives and, moreover, relationships. Over the years, secrets, alliances, and little conspiracies lend shape to relationships. The sparks of an earlier divorce and remarriage often rekindle during illness and revive old hurts and old alliances. Strategic announcing then fits into that history and, likely, continues it.

Given such relationships, others might think that what the ill person says is a strategic announcement even when he or she meant it as a disclosure of information. In a troubled relationship, for example, the ill person may delay disclosing because he or she hesitates to introduce more problems into a continuing saga of conflict. But others view the delay differently. They might see it as a strategic ploy to keep them unaware and to maintain power. To illustrate: when a middle-aged man's heart condition worsened, he told his second wife and older son by his first marriage, but he delayed telling his younger son. After years of anger and conflict, he no longer knew how to talk with this son. When his son learned that everyone else knew several months before he did, he felt that his father had cheated him again. To him, the delay symbolized his father's power and testified to his low status in the family.

The logical extension of making strategic announcements is flaunting illness. When people flaunt illness, they extend further control over their audience and try to extract a specific response, often shock or guilt, from them. These people use their illness in a strategic performance, complete with acting, timing, and staging. I was party to such a performance while interviewing a middle-aged social worker about some of her patients. When I arrived for the interview, she was seated behind her desk; a bulky sweater, thrown over her shoulders, covered her arms. She told me to take the seat directly in front of her desk. Her left hand rested on the desk and her right hand on her lap. After a few minutes of discussing the patients, she announced that her husband had committed suicide on Christmas Eve the year before. Then, she looked me in the eye, smiled malevolently, lifted her right arm out from underneath the sweater, placed it conspicuously on the desk, and waited expectantly for my response. I ignored the fact that she had no hand. She seemed surprised that I was not. I did feel that I had ruined her show. The last scene had not gone according to cue; the performance failed. At that point, she rather grumpily told me that she had diabetes with complications.

At least during the performance, people who flaunt illness seem to separate their present self, experience, and feelings about illness from their portrayal of it. Thus, they objectify self and illness and treat them as products that they manipulate for audience effect.

Paradoxically, however, people may flaunt illness or disability again and again because they feel immersed in it and angry about it. Sometimes they resent everyone else because they feel so diminished by illness and disability. If so, their feelings may assume an objective, staged face as they flaunt their illness.

Plans for Disclosing

Developing a plan for disclosing allows an individual to protect self, others, and relationships. Often, ill people do not intend to avoid disclosing. But, they want to prepare themselves for it. Their plans turn on *what* they disclose and *how* they disclose it.

Softening the news teaches others a tempered view of illness. Like professionals, ill people soften the news by stressing the positive, by glossing over any dark feelings, and by claiming an active stance toward their treatment. Hence, they soften the impact of their news by trying to balance it. Softening the news to others can give ill people the strength to deal with it. These disclosures indicate how people try to soften their news:

> I have a chronic illness; I have MS, but my doctor thinks I'll have a benign course.
> The doctor says I had a heart attack; it had to be minor, because I hardly felt anything.
> I'm having another flare-up and have to go on prednisone, but I know what to expect and it is a matter of riding it out.

Softening the news alters the content of ill people's disclosures. For example, rather than giving her sister the full story, Marty Gordon said, "I tiptoe around it; I don't tell her much."

Similarly, separating feelings from the news transforms disclosing into informing. The content changes. Ill people leave out their sorrow, anger, or remorse. By separating emotion from information, they control how others perceive them, their information, and, moreover, their emotions. As a woman with cancer stated, "I can tell somebody something very serious. I'm pleasant, unflappable, funny, and in control. I can tell them that I have fifteen positive lymph nodes. . . . When I don't pour out all this emotion, I feel more in control."

By managing her emotions, this same woman also managed the meaning of her news and thus reduced its threat (cf. Pearlin 1989). Separating emotion from information gives respite from and control over a flood of emotions, while minimizing the chance of eliciting another's sorrow, shock, or pity. The subsequent strength that these people feel provides continuity with their earlier selves. Occasionally, moreover, they may even discover that they have more strength than they thought they had. In contrast to Hochschild's (1983) argument against suppressing feelings, illness provides one context in which separating emotion from interaction can have positive consequences.[3] Doing so conserves energy and preserves consistency of self.

Structuring protective disclosures includes using the following four strategies: 1) invoking the assistance of others, 2) setting the stage, 3) providing progressive clues, and 4) selective informing. Invoking the assistance of others buttresses both the message and the scene. Assistants can then help keep the scene together, if not the individual participants. Further, someone else's presence usually reflects a unified view and a statement of their shared relationship. For example, when a woman told her former in-laws about her illness, she took her new husband with her. A gay man took his lover, whom his parents hated, with him when he told them about his cancer. Couples together told their children because as Patricia Kennedy said, "This is a family illness—it affects everyone."

Invoking the assistance of professionals, especially physicians, makes the information real and legitimate to others. Since her husband saw her as hypochondriacal, a woman with heart disease wanted to ensure that he had exactly the same information that she had. Unable to tell his wife about receiving a grim prognosis, a man with lymphoma asked his physician to do it.

A long, but undiagnosed, illness can lead to methodical plans for disclosing the overdue diagnosis if family and friends have long discounted an ill person as an authentic and reliable adult. For example, a woman's doctors hospitalized her again for symptoms that everyone, including herself, believed were psychologically induced. When told that she had a bona fide illness, she took special care in telling her husband. For some time, he had accused her of fabricating symptoms and had left the relationship, but not the house, for another woman. Given her strained marriage, this woman enlisted her specialist's aid in disclosing to her husband. She wanted the specialist to underscore the validity of her complaints. Simultaneously, she hoped that having her husband acknowledge her symptoms as legitimate might change his attitude toward her and establish a new emotional climate in the household.

A supportive professional adds reassurance as well as reality to the disclosure. Patricia Kennedy recalled, "The pediatrician came down and said, 'and it's important for you to tell your children this, that you're not going to die and to reassure them and to keep reassuring them.' So the pediatrician was very helpful; he spoke with both the kids privately, and said he felt they were okay, but it was just that we all needed time to get used to it, not just me."

Certainly a doctor's office sets the stage for making announcements. But ill people also can create a stage for imparting news. They plan the "right" kind of setting and ambiance for easing a relative or friend into the disclosure. Like physicians, they may plan to tell the other person in a private place without interruption. These people usually plan to disclose directly, face to face, so they can see the other person's response rather than making a possibly disruptive phone call.

Concern with staging intensifies when ill people decide that they must disclose everything at one time. They must disclose before someone else does it—either inadvertently or intentionally—and before physical changes become visible. A history of misunderstandings or accumulated "wrongs" done to the other person also prompts ill people to stage their disclosures carefully. Handling the disclosure well helps to set the record straight and shows respect for the other person. Thus, frequently, ill people make more detailed plans for disclosing to someone with whom they have had a conflicted, even distant, relationship than to others for whom they have had much more unreserved affection. For example, an older woman told all the other members of her family of her recurrence of cancer except one daughter. She said, "I want to tell Sally [her daughter] in the right way; I can't just call up and drop this one on her. It's harder to tell Sally than the rest of the family because there's been tension between us. So I've been thinking about how I'll do it. She's so busy especially at this time of year. But I think I should talk with her when we won't be interrupted. I'll just invite her over for coffee and tell her when there are just the two of us here."

Planning not only helped her control the disclosure, but also protected the emotions each felt about it.

Providing progressive clues complements staging (Glaser and Strauss 1965). Over time, the ill person gives hints, warnings, and information to someone else. If the other individual already knows about the illness without realizing its progression, the ill person builds on the seriousness of it. For example, a woman who finished chemotherapy mentioned, "I'm feeling terrific since I got off the chemotherapy. All my tests are fine and the doctors are really pleased. It's looking good. The oncologist did say that it is possible to have micro-metastases in cases like mine." By mentioning the possibility of micro-metastases, she reminded her audience that her recovered health may not be assured.

Long past, rather than present, crises, such as having had a heart attack, pose other problems. Family and friends can forget or ignore these illnesses and their residual disabilities. Subsequently, some people with invisible conditions toss reminders to select others that they live with the nagging threat of further illness. They wish to impart such messages as, "I may not look sick, but I am sick," or "I live with the possibility of a crisis developing anytime." Then, in the event of further or sudden illness, family and friends are not caught by surprise.

Hence, these little disclosures define illness as still part of the present and future, not simply the past.

Providing progressive clues often depends on selective informing, which allows ill people to acknowledge certain aspects of their illness, but to minimize others, in order to protect their friends, and often, themselves, as well. People use selective informing when they believe that others need to know something about their illness, but not everything. They push for an immediate doctor's appointment but do not reveal how frightened they feel. They discuss symptoms but evade giving suspected diagnoses. They disclose a diagnosis, but not the prognosis. Later, they can offer more progressive, more serious clues should they need to. In addition, if their condition suddenly worsens, others can make some sense of it. Marty Gordon recounted what she told her husband after her doctor's appointment:

When I finally saw Dr. Ziegler he said, "We're in trouble with your hands; you have gangrene." I said, "I guess I'd figured that." [After the examination], Gary [her husband] said immediately, "What did he say about your hands?" "Oh, he said they'll start clearing up." "Well, what did he say you should do?" "Well nothing much." [To me]: I really kind of low-keyed that.

Selective informing achieves three other major purposes. First, it allows ill people to preserve the earlier structure of the relationship, and subsequently maintain their autonomy and independence. Thus, an elderly woman tells her daughter, who lives in another state, about her hospitalization—not about her occasional falls and dizzy spells. This woman avoids a family crisis about whether she should live alone and maintains her relationship with her daughter as it had been in the past.

Second, selective informing enables ill people to believe that they ease another person's strain. Their decisions about what, when, and how to disclose turn on their assessments of this individual's life. For example, Bessie Thompkins told her daughter, Elsie, about the tests her doctor had scheduled but decided not to tell her about her increasing chest pains, despite describing Elsie as her "best friend." Elsie had three teen-agers still at home, a grandson to babysit, and a husband who had just had a triple bypass operation. Bessie said, "Walter [her son-in-law] isn't handling it very well either. And Elsie's already got so much to do. My daughter's got two babies to take care of so she doesn't need me telling her things that will just make her worry more."

Third, selective informing sets the stage for later concern or assistance without overusing them prematurely. Single and older people often struggled to maintain their independence long after their physicians told them that they should not live alone. For example, a single, middle-aged woman selectively disclosed information to her only relative, a brother, with whom she had shared a cordial, though not close, relationship. She had occasionally socialized with her brother and his family, but neither she nor her brother had ever relied on each other. Their lives had taken different paths, his with his business and family, hers with her secretarial job and a small circle of friends. She felt that she should not expect much present or future help from him. Moving in with them would affect his family, especially since the youngest boy would have to give up his bedroom. Her past relationship with the family, and the amount of disability she had already experienced, influenced her decision to carefully meter information to them. Hence, she tried to preserve their past relationship without burdening them with her presence or with future obligations.

Selective informing can strain relationships, however, when the provided information insufficiently accounts for an ill individual's behavior. Bonnie Presley had told her twenty-two-year-old daughter little about how lupus erythematosus had affected her life. Upon returning home to live with her again after five years, her daughter confronted her about her limited activities. Bonnie explained:

> Last Friday a week ago, we just really had words. She finally—I don't know what happened; I don't know what started it. She said, "Mommy, I just can't take this anymore; you never go anywhere; you never do anything; you know, you're just staying home all the time and—" I said, "Hey, this is all I can do, you

know. I'm trying to better myself, and I'm reading but I don't have the energy that you remember." 'Cause see, when she left me—left me, went away; I hadn't seen her for a couple years, I was working out, working full time—she used to call me the bionic woman. . . . Then when I explained it to her, everything's been real good. She said, "Why didn't you tell me?"

6

Living with Chronic Illness

I've gone through twelve weeks of cardiac rehabilitation and they gave me a daily chart that I'm supposed to continue. I'm supposed to do back exercises and the cardiac exercises . . . and then I'm supposed to walk for thirty to forty-five minutes each day. When I do, sometimes I might walk for an hour but I haven't done it this last week—it was hot to begin with and I didn't go out and I didn't exercise and then I've been having so much trouble with my back, and I get dizzy when I lay down on the floor [to exercise].

I was frustrated for so long with the asthma, not being able to do things and then the bowel problem came along. . . . What it does to your nerves [laughs ruefully] is terrible.

If we are going anywhere like on a hike, and we leave early the next day so the night before, I'll take four or five pills for the bowel so I don't have to have a bowel [movement] and then I just don't eat anything after 6:00 and then I am real careful about what I eat so that I can plan ahead to do this thing. So it gets hard. . . . You have to stop and think before you make something—you've got to put a little more time into it.

From embarrassment to mortification. From discomfort to pain. Endless uncertainty. What follows? Regimentation. Ann Rorty, a fifty-four-year-old woman, spent her days minimizing pain and avoiding humiliation. Planning, scheduling, and timing absorbed her thoughts. Frustration and anxiety resulted when her efforts failed. Ann found herself in midlife with asthma, chronic back pain, bowel incontinence and, most recently, heart disease. Her varied conditions with their respective regimens contradicted each other. If she followed her surgeon's advice to treat her back pain with bed rest, she interrupted her cardiac exercise regimen. If she ate a healthy diet for her heart, she caused havoc with her intestine. If she could return to work, her morale would improve but her back pain would worsen since she could not stand or sit for long.

How do people like Ann Rorty handle daily life? What can people with multiple chronic conditions do to preserve and continue their independence? How do they plan to avoid embarrassment and humiliation? What is it like to follow stringent diets, rigid schedules, and unusual treatments? How, if at all, do ill people create and handle strange new routines?

In Chapter 3, I discussed keeping illness contained as a strategy to maintain continuity of self. In this chapter, I show how living with illness merges with strategies to keep illness contained.

Contexts of Life

Living with chronic illness occurs within social and personal contexts including the structure of medical care. As a result, the problems of living with illness fall squarely on ill people and by extension, their families and friends (Conrad 1985; Corbin and Strauss 1988; Gerhardt and Brieskorn-Zinke 1986; Locker 1983; Schneider and Conrad 1983; Strauss et al. 1984). As a logical consequence of fragmentation within the medical care system, people commonly handle illness in individualistic, idiosyncratic ways, frequently in isolation and with little information.[1] As a result, ill people become innovators in handling their illnesses, inventors of their lives, and creators of ways of coping. Not surprisingly, some of their inventions remain taken for granted and unnoted. Furthermore, they do not think of other possibilities or realize when they might have choices. Rather, their inventions and adaptations flow together in what eventually feels natural.

Living with chronic illness occurs within a context that includes age, class, gender, occupation, marital status, and type and extent of disability. Age and class affect whether someone's inventions remain taken-for-granted adaptations or explicit strategies. Very old people, especially working- and lower-middle-class elders, likely have long been disconnected from community and society. They adjust and adapt to their plights. Younger individuals, especially well-educated professionals, chafe at such disconnection—or the threat of it—and often devise elaborate strategies to preserve their pursuits and their lives.

Strategies for living with illness change as it progresses. Someone who hid illness later acknowledges it. Someone who once juggled regimens and treatments to conceal illness at work later retires and just keeps it contained during social events. People may abandon elaborate strategies in favor of more simple ones.

Learning to live with illness develops as people form and collect strategies to get through the day and revise them as their conditions change (Jobling 1977; 1988). Their efforts spur questions about the logistics of scheduling, pacing, and handling spatial arrangements. They must take into account the need to follow regimens and control symptoms, as well as all the other logistics of living—caring for children, being sexual, doing housework, cooking, shopping, and keeping a physically or psychologically stressful job.

Many people attend to their illness when it prevents them from remaking their lives or when it immediately impinges upon them. If living with illness and following valued pursuits do not complement each other, people put their pursuits first. Throughout each day, they sacrifice their health in small ways. For example, Heather Robbins was determined to raise her children herself. As a result, she lifted and carried them. She said, "My legs still aren't that strong. And I use my back to lift rather than my legs to lift and it hurts."

Living with illness raises the question: which illness? Chronically ill people often devote their efforts to the most intrusive ailment and minimize a less noticeable one. The possibility of bowel incontinence structured Ann Rorty's daily routine. By remaining at home until the afternoon, she could better discern if she could risk leaving the house at all. Unlike some people, Ann could talk about controlling incontinence. Her heart condition, however, seemed more ambiguous and the consequences of ignoring it more intangible. She commented, "I can't get the heart problem out there where I can deal with it and talk with it, about it, because I don't know what it's going to do or, everything that, you know, surrounds it. I know what diets and the exercise you should do and shouldn't do but like, it's not cut and dry."

For her, living with illness meant predicting her limits of medical noncompliance without causing herself harm. She had to know the size of the container and how it could be wrapped before she could keep her heart condition contained.

Very ill people must learn to plan the minutiae of their lives, if they are to remain independent. A woman with multiple sclerosis found that if things were slightly out of place, she could not manage them. If her sweater was in the bottom dresser drawer instead of the second drawer, she usually lost her balance and fell while trying to pull the drawer open. If the vacuum in the hall closet got caught on the carpet edge while being wheeled out, she could not lift it over the carpet. If the trash got too full or heavy, she might drop it while carrying it out.

Inability to handle routine tasks evokes existential dilemmas about self-worth, living at all, and limitation. Dropping the trash takes on magnified meaning. To the ill person, it means more than miscalculation or clumsiness. It symbolizes a diminished self. Tremendous frustration, anger, and despair result. Consequently, many ill people organize their lives to reduce the number and intensity of such existential glimpses of self and the feelings they invoke.

Changes in people's lives bring different needs. For example, nine years ago, Patricia Kennedy wrestled with the logistics of handling her regimen, doing housework, and chauffering her boys all over the county. Grown children and new goals changed what she needed to do. Her plans to return to work coincided with her oldest son learning to drive. He took over most of the errands. His help allowed her time to work and to rest. Having help provided a buffer for her self-concept and self-esteem.

Remaking a Life

The problems with which ill people struggle are existential; their solutions are often organizational.[2] To remake a life, they need to focus and organize their efforts. They attempt to take control of their lives by organizing time, space, themselves, and other individuals. They ask such questions as: "How can I get through the workday?" "How can I save energy?" "What can I cut out?" Remaking a life includes planning, tightening, and modifying or reorganizing tasks and activities.

Being aware of one's efforts to organize turns on: 1) defining sharp contrasts between before and after the illness, 2) having always noted such efforts, 3) puzzling over how to make innovations, and 4) seeing one's independence threatened. A man who had had a heart attack explained, "I had to change my life; otherwise I wouldn't live."

Of course, an ill person can find it useful to have a set of needs and tasks that must take priority. A middle-aged man said of his regimen of diet, exercise, and rest: "It's my excuse to pamper myself and to put myself first. I've got something now that I have to insist on selflessly. It's not my mind; it's my body."

Not uncommonly, ill individuals organize their activities carefully and methodically without full awareness of why they make certain plans and choices. A woman with cancer wore a cap, which did not cover her hair loss. She did not realize that she tried to avoid embarrassment until she read an earlier draft of this material. She said, "I get out before people are in the streets and walk my dog early in the morning and at dusk because I'm shy about losing my hair."

When someone has always tightly organized activities, schedules, and tasks, illness presents yet another realm of life to plan and manage. Patricia Kennedy commented, "I've always been an organizer—that's how I've gotten things done. I like an orderly life; I like to know what I'm doing and when I need to do it." Once she ordered her life for efficiency and productivity. As her illness progressed, she aimed to limit fatigue, suppress embarrassing symptoms, such as an unsteady gait, and avoid stares and questions. She managed her time and pursuits to preserve a valued self.

Managing a regimen for years, such as a cardiac diet and exercise program, results in it becoming part of daily routine (Davis 1963; Kelleher 1988). A young physician with diabetes did not see himself as attending much to his illness. However, he had perfectly synchronized his busy schedule to fit his illness and regimen and to keep them hidden, although he did not dwell on illness per se. He planned his daily schedule to allow for rest periods, meals, and exercise. Further, he arranged to take his insulin just before or after work and dates. Yet, not until he recounted his regimen did he realize how he had organized it. In contrast, when people's efforts feel bizarre or when they are plagued by continual reminders that they cannot do things the way others do, they know precisely what they organize, why they do it, and how they do it.

Constantly coping with a steadily progressive illness or suffering from an unpredictable condition poses enormous existential and organizational problems. The need for continual reorganizing can drain and discourage ill people. An elderly woman noted, "Just when you think you've got things planned and manageable—*wham*—another complication, more disturbing symptoms and you're back to where you started again."

Organizing tasks can extend through an entire household. Married men draw upon the assistance of their wives. Women often must enlist the aid of children and husbands or companions. A middle-aged woman served as coordinator and overseer of household tasks, but executed none of them. She shifted the burden to her five daughters who took over the housework and to her husband who added the yardwork to his home maintenance duties. Involving other family members enabled this woman to continue to work. Another woman could not do housework because multiple sclerosis had left her arms too weak to reach beyond her wheelchair. Despite her failing eyesight, she could locate everything in the household (Charmaz 1987). She saw herself as the family organizer since everyone depended on her:

I am *organized*—got it from my mother, there is a place for every-thing, a time to do it, a place to wear everything. . . . I keep track of everything that is needed even though my husband does the shopping. I have my desk and keep all the appointments for the children and organize what Mrs. Roberts [her housekeeper] should do each day. [She laughed.] My husband says this place would be chaos if I didn't keep everything straight. (Charmaz 1987:312)

Taking on the role of household organizer reduced this woman's feelings of guilt about "otherwise being a drain on the family."

More frequently, ill women organized some tasks for others to do but continued to do most of the housework themselves. For example, mothers of teen-agers enlisted them to drive and load the car but still cooked and cleaned. Heather Robbins's first serious flare-up of multiple sclerosis occurred when she was a single mother of her little girl, Tammy. Though she felt that she had expected too much from the child, she had discovered that Tammy could help. She said, "She was getting herself dressed at eighteen months. . . . She knew how to open the refrigerator; she got yogurt and food to eat. She would help carry things up the stairs and she was just a baby."

Women, as well as their families, commonly believed that they had to function as before. Several mothers, however, found that allowing time for rest and regimen meant abandoning the "supermom" role. Subsequently, the entire household needed reorganizing. That meant relying upon children and husbands to do unfamiliar tasks. Patricia Kennedy had to teach her son what dust looked like. She said, "I would take him over to a table and point to it and say, 'what's that on the table?'; he would look at it and blink, 'Nothing.' Now he knows what dust looks like and I don't even have to ask him to do the dusting; he just pitches in and it's not a big deal."

Women taught husbands and children how to do the laundry, make beds, and plan meals. Spouses and children who had already been involved *extended* the kinds of work that they had been doing. A woman who had diabetes had always shared household tasks with her husband. Her life-threatening insulin crisis caused him to extend his involvement to organizing and monitoring her care.

Similarly, men also organized tasks but then delegated them to other family members, such as driving, managing business accounts, and maintaining the car. Their efforts allowed them to feel that family life remained under control, even if they could not do the tasks themselves.

Single adults enlisted their parents and siblings in the work. A young woman's sore, stiff joints made getting into clothes a time-consuming daily trauma. She asked her mother to adapt her clothes to her changing body. A sister did grocery shopping and errands for her ill brother. A few single people had relatives who sensed when to help. Gloria Krause's divorced mother came to live with her when she got sicker. Her father and his wife sent money and provided help during their visits.

Yet, family and friends may limit their involvement. Some relatives volunteered to organize help but would not give it, which commonly happened to single elders. Other relatives and friends helped but placed time limits on what they could do. For example, a middle-aged woman's husband helped occasionally with the housework. But they both agreed that keeping up with his business and graduate program came first. Several spouses took over household tasks and childcare but expected their partners to keep working, despite serious illness.

Before becoming ill, many people had not thought about organizing their day. Afterwards, they found it a consuming interest. Immersion in illness makes completing the most basic self-care a major hurdle. As Sara Shaw recalled, "My energy was incredibly low, so I would really organize it [self-care] out [while in bed]. I would have every single little thing down that I needed to do. I would go from one [thing] to the other. Then when I would get up to do it, I wouldn't have to think about it. I would have it organized. I would do exactly what I needed to do then I would be back in bed as soon as the energy went down."

Like others, Sara learned to organize through being ill. She said, "I'm really good about effective use of time now. I learned a lot about that when I was ill. . . . You can just have time go along and be spread out all over the place and not get the things done that are really important. So what's important for me to do at this time? That was learned, conditioned while I was sick."

Another young woman thought through exactly what she would need to do in order to create a life for herself. Before her illness, she had lived spontaneously, following intuition and whim. She described herself as having been someone who would travel three thousand miles on a moment's notice without taking a coat or money. Afterwards, she planned her life— from developing stable friendships to solidifying her finances and choosing a favorable climate—before she reentered a university. She said, "The first year I was trying to decide just what I wanted to do. The second two years I was saving money and actually making up little shoe repair kits. I just organized my whole life—my files. Instead of having things all over, I had a shoe repair care kit, a box with ribbons and papers, plant care kit, every single thing in my life is organized."

This woman not only reorganized her belongings for accessibility and convenience, she organized a life that would aid her in reaching her goals. In that way, she improved her chances of living on her own terms. Moreover, she planned a foundation on which she could build a valued self.

Illness also can prompt the further development of organizational skills. An older woman with lupus knew that she could not handle the rigors of an office job. Like many lupus patients, she also shielded herself from the sun. By creating her own business and working at home, she avoided the relentless sun in her hot valley town and paced her day so that she could take rest periods. By working in a darkened room, she protected her health and, moreover, organized a manageable job.

Learning effective organization depends upon fitting activities between hopes and plans. This often means scaling down hopes and former expectations of self and planning around disability. Even though psychologist Ernest A. Hirsch's disability benefit provided a comfortable income, he continued to work without pay, since work structured his life. He observes, "Coming to work every day gives a certain body to my life and prevents it from flowing away in a formless puddle. Work gives me something to look forward to and to look backward on, a tomorrow, a now and a yesterday that organizes and shapes" (1977:134).

Reconciling hopes and plans affects the organization of each day. Being supermom had structured Patricia Kennedy's self-concept and daily life. However, having multiple sclerosis forced her to plan around her disability. She anticipated the amount of activity that she could handle and realized that doing more accelerated her fatigue and discomfort. "I always prepare for evening activities. I always take a two-hour nap in the afternoon, even if I'm not tired."

Making Tradeoffs

When ill people try to organize their lives, they weigh and measure what they can do and the importance of doing it; they make trade-offs.[3] Their choices, tacit adaptations, and unwitting changes reveal their trade-offs. Which trade-offs do they make, and how do they do they make them? They simplify their lives, reorder their time, and juggle and pace their activities to fit their lives.

Simplifying Life

Simplifying means eliminating some events, activities, and tasks entirely, and reducing the steps, obstacles, complexities, and necessary time and space of others. Although simplifying reduces effort and stress, the costs come in the trade-offs— forced trade-offs. Ill people assess their physical stamina and survey their daily tasks. "What can I give up?" "How can I make things easier?"

Simplifying preserves the most necessary activities by making them easier. Including others in a task simplifies it and simultaneously maintains the social relationship. Patricia Kennedy said, "With David's [her husband] schedule, I don't plan things like real elaborate meals during the week because I never know when he is going to leave the office. So rather than putting an additional stress on me, I don't start to cook until he comes. We cook together; it is a good time for us you know, we can talk, catch up on what's happened during the day. It's a real good time and I wonder why we didn't do this all along."

Here, Patricia Kennedy gained doubly, for she shared social space as well as the task. Similarly, Heather Robbins lay down when she nursed her baby so that she could rest a bit. Simplifying tasks allows the person to continue to do them, and at the same time also saves energy for other pursuits. Carolyn Hardesty writes, "My dearest aunt sent me an electric can opener since I could not grip the handles of a manual one with enough force to puncture a lid. We switched from cloth to paper diapers because I couldn't open or shut a safety pin. . . . I made a rare visit to a hair salon for a permanent so my hair would take care of itself after a quick shampoo in the shower (this I could do only be easing my arms up, never elbows out)" (1987:21).

Added responsibilities blur simplifying for illness. For example, having a child or getting a full-time job force most parents to reorganize their lives and to simplify some tasks. After her second child was born, Heather Robbins occupied her toddler with television programs to give herself some respite. She also discovered that having another baby legitimated simplifying her social involvements:

> It's easy for me to say, "I have a baby; I don't have to do this"—if somebody's planning a lot of—something that takes a lot of walking, hiking, or something that maybe I just can't do. . . . We'll go places that we know we can take it easy. I can lay down with him [baby]. Where she [toddler] can run around and play and do things like that, but I don't have to be running around like a chicken with my head cut off planning a lot of things. We don't have a lot of dinner parties, not that we had that many anyway. I mean we had company over like twice a week; they were like hot rods and we just don't do it anymore. It's easier not to.

Changes, compromises, and sacrifices permit ill people to carry on a life, albeit a simplified one (cf. Reif 1975). That's the trade-off. A middle-aged single woman read novels she didn't like because she could still get to the supermarket where she bought them. She traded reading bad novels for risking the embarrassment of asking someone to go to the library for her. Elderly people ate TV dinners rather than prepare meals. Many people who did cook fixed enough food for several days or a week. They traded variety for convenience. Christine Danforth kept her job and her bowling league's records, and simplified everything else. She said, "As it is now, I wash the dishes once a week; I rinse them and throw them on the counter and then, just wash them [later]; it's easier."

When possible, other people trade expense for services. After he inherited money, Mark Reinertsen eliminated cooking by eating one hot meal at a restaurant each day. Chronically ill elders, who lived alone but had financial resources, hired help for tasks they used to do themselves. (Similarly, working people buy services and thereby gain time for work or rest.) After several years of living marginally, Bonnie Presley started an accounting business. She remarked, "I have a housekeeper now and I have my nails done every week. I don't do my ironing; I don't clean my house. She does the laundry; I do my personal laundry, but she does all the other laundry. And I really can't afford it but I do it anyway. Because there's no way I can go work all day and come home and clean and stuff. So I made that choice too. And the business is just going to have to pay for it."

Occasionally, people will simplify their homes by ridding them of extra furniture, knick-knacks, and accumulated remnants of the past. They close off unneeded rooms, move their bedroom downstairs, or add a bathroom. This allows them to move about with greater efficiency, control, and, often, safety. Other people rid themselves of their homes. A middle-aged divorced woman with heart disease sold her home and rented an apartment, which she shared with her nearly blind aged mother. She traded privacy for efficiency and for closer monitoring of her mother's health. She thereby eliminated yardwork, reduced housework, and streamlined her daily schedule. Previously she had cleaned, cooked, and cared for her mother in addition to managing her own health and household.

People develop different ways to simplify their lives. Few people can remodel their homes. Not everyone thinks of using space in new or easier ways. But many people revise their standard of living downward. John Garston said, "I don't have to exert myself all that much and am able to maintain something [do enough work] where I eat. It is, you know, a low standard of living."

Standards of cleanliness and housekeeping also slide downward. Vera Mueller remarked, "My house has never been clean. I never have had the physical stamina to do everything. And the minute one thing gets clean, something else gets dirty."

Not surprisingly, the trade-offs in housekeeping prey more on women's minds than on men's. Tina Reidel kept her job, followed her spiritual path, and took time for herself. But she did not clean the house, which she saw as one of her "deficiencies." She added:

> And then the house, I think I feel all stressed out when I come home, 'cause it's such a—you know, I'm a pack rat and it's a mess and then I get all stressed out when I come home, 'cause the house looks like some part of my pysche that I don't want to deal with. Like it's chaos and all the beautiful things in the house—like in my room are strewn all over the place. I don't want to deal with them. The physical is like sort of tearing at me and I don't want to spend my physical energy to fix up the house. Like whenever I have some energy, I want to spend it on myself [giggles]. It's like I'm so limited. 'Cause I'm always trying to do stuff for the self. . . . So it's almost like to balance all that stuff [being in pain].

If no one else can or will do household tasks, they remain undone. Unkept houses lead to embarrassment and simplifying further by eliminating visitors. A single woman took much pride in remaining independent but couldn't bear to have guests. She remarked, "I'm independent but my cottage is a wreck."

Gradual erosion of prior standards of household or personal cleanliness usually occurs imperceptibly. When depressed, isolated, and ill, people's standards of cleanliness fade. Also, some older people can not see the dirt and cobwebs. An elderly husband's illness had become both preoccupation and occupation for him and his wife. After her unexpected death, he seemed unaware of grime and clutter. He simplified unwittingly. He did almost as little as he had before her death and began to drink heavily. Certainly grief, loneliness, depression, and disorientation can contribute to such responses, whether from dislocation, disconnection, drug interactions, or drunkeness.

People not only simplify self-care and household tasks, they also simplify hobbies. That way they can still follow valued pusuits. Nancy Swenson stated:

> I'm not going to quit on the garden; I'm just going to make it smaller. . . . I'm going to simplify it and experiment and I think it's going to be kind of neat, because I'm going to make planter boxes with wire under it to keep the gophers out and I'm only going to have certain things. You know, just enough for the family and make more variety. And something so it won't be a lot of work. . . . I think people need, when they're ill, to do something that's rewarding, to make them feel good about themselves. . . . Look at this tomato, I mean I was proud—I mean I had some beautiful tomatoes. And I think you need that. You need some free self-esteem.

As health decreases, self-care takes precedence and activities shrink to a bare minimum (Fagerhaugh 1975). Hence, ill people will trade efficiency for being able to function at all. A middle-aged woman shopped at an expensive neighborhood market because she could park in front of the door and purchase basic supplies by making one round through the small store. But she couldn't get any other errands done simultaneously. If she shopped at the supermarket, however, she could also buy household items, refill prescriptions, and go to the post office. When she went to the neighborhood store, she lost efficiency because she had to do more time-consuming errands later; but in another sense, she gained it by avoiding exhaustion.

Performing one major task a day helped many ill people to manage their care. For example, to simplify his day and to preserve his energy, a retired man scheduled no more than one main event in a day, such as a doctor's appointment. A woman commented, "I try to do one hard thing each day—I grocery shop one day, cook another, and do the laundry another so that I don't get so exhausted."

Most people think about ways to simplify certain tiring tasks—such as shopping, cooking, and cleaning. Elderly people often shopped when the stores first opened because of light traffic, empty aisles, and short lines. A streamlined route without delays simplified their task (Fagerhaugh 1975). Determining the quickest and most convenient way to complete a task helped cut steps. Nancy Swenson said:

> I find cooking real easy; I've learned a lot of tricks since I've been ill. . . . And a lot of what of I do is—is I cook a large amount of some things . . . and then freeze [portions]. Well, from start to finish, I can have a healthy meal on the table in half an hour. . . . I'll take a pot roast and I'll cook it in the crockpot with potatoes and carrots and that's a meal. Well then what's left of the pot roast . . . I put back in the crockpot and . . . add maybe a can of chili con carne . . . and mix this up, and get some flour tortillas and cut up some tomatoes . . . and just heat up a tortilla at a time. . . . So [next] I make a beef soup out of it [the remaining leftovers] with the stock and the gravy. I thin it down and then I just start adding all kinds of vegetables and maybe a little pasta. . . . And then I'll get a loaf of French bread and we've got our meat and our vegetables and a healthy meal there. . . .
>
> So I find cooking—cooking is just a snap, you know. You just—I guess you learn these things when you're sick and you don't feel good. You learn these little shortcuts. I remember entertaining and preparing so far ahead and working so hard and now, you know, I can put things together and they're just as healthy and just as good, and sometimes even better in just no time at all.

Simplified self-care that begins in the aftermath of a crisis can last far longer than ill people had anticipated. Financial and physical strain can make it necessary to continue a "temporary" adaptation. For example, a middle-aged woman who had prided herself on her fastidious appearance had to relinquish her grooming due to a medical crisis. Later, she had no choice. She could not apply her makeup neatly; nor could she afford the costs of dry cleaning and hair coloring. She had to accept as permanent what had been temporary measures during a difficult period. Her range of possible trade-offs narrowed considerably. For her, a temporary present became a permanent future.

Staying home is a major strategy for managing illness (Locker 1983). Why leave the house at all if going anywhere is so difficult? Leaving the house means work. Planning uncongested routes. Arranging rides. Getting help. Packing supplies. Organizing medications. Ironing a shirt or dress. Added to the work are all the "what if's?": "What if my bladder leaks?" "What if they don't serve anything I can eat?" "What if my hand starts to shake during dinner?" "What if I get into trouble in public?" By staying home, ill people can jettison both public self-presentation and the preparation that it entails. By shrinking space, they expand units of time. Moreover, poor people as well as those who cannot drive are forced to stay home. John Garston said, "I literally don't leave here. I garden and eat out of my garden. . . . I'm stuck here." An elderly woman who suffered from urinary incontinence said, "I don't leave the house anymore; it is just easier than taking all that paraphernalia and risking being mortified anyway. It is just too embarrassing." As a result of her illness, Patricia Kennedy had reorganized her home. She remarked, "Home is a real safe environment because I have it set up so that everything is convenient. It is a very safe place and leaving it is scary."

A simplified life at home feels safe due to its familiarity and predictability. Staying home means less anxiety and distress, and therefore fewer existential confrontations. Nonetheless, even if one remains at home, the existential questions of meaning, purpose, and productivity in life can persist and increase.

Tacitly or even explicitly, ill people sometimes simplify tasks as a trade-off for maintaining significant relationships. They may abbreviate their self-care, or strip their homes of clutter, for the benefit of their caregivers. For example, an elderly woman reluctantly agreed to stop wearing underpants since they caused her husband so much difficulty when he helped her on and off the toilet.

Quite clearly, determining when, how, for whom, and for which purposes to simplify can cause conflicts in families. Such trade-offs are hard won. Conflicts over trade-offs escalate when participants' self-concepts, rather than mere logistics, are at issue, however tacitly that occurs. To several men, accepting hospital beds, commodes, or disposable pads symbolized greater dependence and debility than their self-concepts allowed. They tried to maintain their former dominant roles in the household and to mask their growing physical dependence by barking orders to their wives. They felt that using the equipment compromised their authority and proclaimed frailty and loss.

Caregivers' self-concepts also get caught up in strategies for simplification. What may simplify life for the ill one may mean more work for the caregiver. An elderly woman carefully scheduled only one errand a day, but her daughter had to organize and do that errand. The daughter said, "I have to drive ten miles in heavy traffic to do one thing."

Ill people often simplify by getting or letting someone else do the work or provide the care. Pressures to do so may become overwhelming. The trade-off may be implicit, like being allowed to continue living in one's own apartment. An elderly man refused to use disposable pads for his growing urinary incontinence, which resulted in stacks of laundry and soiled floors. He relented about having his home health worker help him after the visiting nurse insisted that he wear the pads and his daughter threatened to put them on him herself. His nurse and daughter overruled him; they discounted his wishes for modesty in favor of simplifying what had resulted in arduous, unpleasant work.

As a simplified routine grows familiar, it seems normal to the ill person but perhaps bizarre to others. Thus, isolated and depressed ill people "normalize" wearing dirty clothes, living in pajamas, and bathing infrequently (Wiener 1975).[4] In addition, over time, other people normalize seemingly strange simplified routines that help them to function. For example, having attendant care simplified Ernest A. Hirsch's day and allowed him to continue to work:

> It's interesting, in fact, how many things are adapted to, things, which at first may seem altogether strange. One of these changes, which I viewed with dread before I actually undertook it, turned out to be quite easily adapted to. This activity involved having

myself washed, combed, shaved, and so on, rather than doing it myself as I had done practically all my life . . . but since I returned from the hospital in the spring of 1973, I no longer had either the strength or the ability to handle these very personal tasks. Instead, I've asked my live-in helper to add this duty to his others. We have the procedure down to such a science that, from the time I get up in the morning until I appear at the breakfast able, only about three-quarters of an hour elapses. (1977:121)

Tangible symbols of simplifying include moving to a one-story home in an "adult" housing development, eliminating entertaining guests, and deciding to use a handicapped parking spot. However, with each change may come unwelcome symbols of loss and of self as well as chosen trade-offs.

Vivid symbols result from sharply defined categories and shared understandings. Using a wheelchair, for example, symbolizes taking on an identity as seriously disabled. Jean Stewart's crutches caused much difficulty: "Three full years of this nonsense with crutches lay ahead, before I would begin to accept the idea of using a wheelchair. That wheelchairs could be thought of as conveniences rather than as portable prisons, or worse, badges of moral capitulation, was a life-transforming concept that simply did not occur to me" (1987:131).[5]

An appliance that simplifies logistical problems and arduous tasks can confound self-image and social identity. Hence, some ill people prefer to stay at home or to risk heart failure, a fall, or exhaustion rather than use a walker, a wheelchair, or a handicapped parking space. A first indication that they need help can occur when ill people try to make their way through large parking lots or international airports. Mark Reinertsen said, "I went to the Grateful Dead concert and had to park way out. I had to stop three times going across the lot and really didn't know if I'd make it. That really bothered me." Ill people may simplify their homes, reconstruct their routines, and reroute themselves, but they cannot exert similar control over the distances in a parking lot or an airport. They need help.

Using a wheelchair or a cane are ways of simplifying that people remember and may discuss. Other ways of simplifying can remain more hidden—sometimes by intent, but more likely because they become a part of life. For example, a young woman distanced herself from co-workers to avoid becoming involved in their time-consuming chatter during work and tiring social events after work. An older man feigned more confusion than he felt when he received requests that he wanted to refuse. A middle-aged teacher discouraged student contact and demands through sullen looks and sharp retorts. Of course, people may have perfected such tactics long before any chronic illness affected them.

What begins as a way to simplify life can result in later problems, dilemmas, and stresses. Here, the trade-offs do not work. Moving closer to work to avoid a lengthy commute can result in losing contact with friends, as several people discovered who had no time or energy to make new friends. Seeking relief from the stress of city life by moving to the country can produce boredom, relentless poverty, and no medical coverage, as several other people found. Living at an easy pace in retirement may end when money gets tight as an older woman discovered when her life savings evaporated after one medical crisis. Maintaining a shared living arrangement becomes tenuous when health fails, rent climbs, and income dwindles, as the woman who lived with her mother discovered. Reducing work hours can lead to constant worry about money and independence, as a number of people found.

Reordering Time and Scheduling

"What should be my first priority?" "Should I plan to cut back my work hours?" "How can I fit rest periods into the day?" Whether or not to schedule, what to reorder, and when to do it bring ill people face to face with the trade-offs they will make; their existential dilemmas become clearer. Most ill people who work must make trade-offs between time commitments. However, it does not always occur to them to negotiate their scheduling needs, or they may lack the power to do so. In addition, some ill people sometimes schedule for their maximum level of functioning, without taking the questions above into account. They attempt to fit themselves into other people's schedules or an organizational one. When these people cannot function at their maximum level, or meet the organizational schedule, they withdraw entirely. Later, a few of these individuals begin to make trade-offs, if they discover that doing so might afford them more control over their lives.

Trade-offs in reordering and scheduling the day develop in three ways. First, when illness permits, people meld time for illness into an already scheduled day. They extend or adapt their schedules to include illness. Second, when illness worsens, they feel forced to change their lives, and develop "healthier" routines. Third, when ominous warnings develop, people may create or revise their schedules to handle illness. As a man with diabetes recalled:

> I became much more aware of the possibilities of schedules because I had a part-time job; I had classes; I needed to write papers and I had to get exercise. I tried to get up at the same time everyday so that I would take my shot at the same time everyday and so therefore I tried to go to bed at the same time everyday. It was a big change, yeah, before that I just stayed up until I fell asleep; I got very little sleep. I never thought about exercise.

Thus, chronic illness can result in creating a structured routine when none had existed previously. For some people, the need to schedule means facing what they had heretofore dismissed or ignored. But new or renewed awareness of one's vulnerability can prompt scheduling a regimen. The man above said, "You know before, I never noticed what I was eating, or *if* I was eating. It never was of concern to me. It was as though I didn't have—it was as though my *self* didn't extend to the person who ate. I would eat, you know, if there were someone around and they put some food on the table, I would eat it. Otherwise, I wouldn't bother."

People alter their schedules multiple times, as illness, life, or self changes, even subtle or minor changes. For a schedule to work, the person has to link it to preservation of the self as well as the body. A fragile balance of the schedule reflects fragile health. As one woman said,

If I don't sleep well, I drag the whole next day. If I'm dragging, then I don't feel like doing my exercise. Then if I don't do my exercise, I usually don't sleep well again. If I am tired, I don't stop at the store and I don't cook much. Then I don't eat well. With that kind of fatigue, I can't do everything I need to do, so things pile up and everything is slower. And if, on top of it, I get a cold or flu, then my schedule is just shot for weeks.

Here, slots in a schedule stack upon each other like dominoes; one slip and the entire schedule collapses, and with it, cumulative effects on health.[6]

Generally, as noted earlier, time conflicts between work or family demands and a medical regimen get resolved in favor of the former. Furthermore, someone may not have transferred earlier work or family timeframes to suitable timeframes for illness. For example, Ann Rorty retained the timeframe of work long after her physician insisted that she take time off for surgery. Granting high priority to work—and the lack of any sick leave—provide powerful incentives to remain at work, despite ill health. Ann recalled:

He [the doctor] wanted to do an emergency surgery, because he didn't know what the lump was. . . . Well, I told him, "Dr. Brown," I said, "I can't go in right now because I don't have anyone to take my place at work. . . ." All my jobs, you know, I've always been that way. And with us down at Oscar's [a fast-food restaurant], after I became night cook, there was no one to take over. . . . It was just putting a lot of stress on me because I wasn't—I couldn't—I didn't feel like I could just walk away from it. And another thing, we don't get paid for being sick.

Reordering timeframes to account for illness may be disallowed. People who had no sick leave or who had used it up usually lost their jobs. Christine Danforth described a factory where she had worked: "There was no such thing as sick leave or anything like that, so you know, you went to work sick or not. I went to work a lot of times and I was really useless. The women that I work[ed] with are really good and they covered for me. . . . The bosses didn't care, I mean it was like, if you were sick, you needed to die first before you [could take off]."

More commonly, ill people who disregard doctor's orders trade later damage for a present schedule. For example, despite her physician's warnings, a woman increased her medication so that she could work a few hours each day even though doing so accelerated her deteriorating health.

Active men and women often resist scheduling for illness and treatment since trade-offs for illness attest to the reality of it (Speedling 1982). Six years ago, Vera Mueller felt that she had to have more regular meals, rest, exercise, and medical examinations. She said, "It makes me mad. Nobody else has to follow such a strict routine, why should *I?*"

One of the main reasons for reordering time is to schedule timeouts for rest (Skevington 1986). When people work for large organizations, finding ways to rest requires some ingenuity. One woman took long bathroom breaks; another worked quickly in the mornings and shuffled papers in the afternoon when she became tired. Having a supervisory position helps tremendously. A woman said, "I just tell my employees that I have a project to finish and do not want to be disturbed. Then I go lay down on the couch in my office."

Reordering time and scheduling frequently involve working around or within other people's schedules, sometimes fitting illness into their schedules—visits to doctors, help with treatments, etc. When a caregiver is also ill, he or she squeezes self-care into the less demanding times in the other's schedule. For several years, Nancy Swenson tried to rest, do housework, complete forms, and run errands from 10:30 to 1:30, three times a week. These short intervals occurred between delivering and picking up her mother at the Alzheimer's Respite Center.

Commonly, family members must work, attend school, care for children, and so on. An ill relative's schedule can flood their daily round. For example, a middle-aged man felt drowsy when he finished his thrice-weekly dialysis treatments at 12:30 A.M. Though his wife rose before dawn to get ready for work, she routinely picked him up after his treatments. Such added demands can easily exceed the energy of someone who also has a serious chronic illness. Ann Rorty tried to handle her elderly mother's care in addition to her own illnesses, an arduous job, a demanding partner, and her grandchildren's psychological problems. After several months, she turned her mother's care over to a daughter-in-law.

Reordering time *because* of illness can result in reordering time *for* family and friends. Several middle-aged men realized that before their illness, work had consumed them. Afterwards, they refused to let their work, and sometimes their illness as well, to interfere with family time. After his heart attack, five years ago, a businessman changed his schedule so that he could spend evenings and weekends with his family rather than working as he had for the previous twenty-five years. He said:

> I'm not as dedicated to the company as I was prior to my surgery. I have more of a family dedication and I hope they never hear that. . . . If the company were—happened to be done with you, they cut the ties and that's it; it's all over with. And there would be somebody else the following day to take your place and I—I really cherish the time with my family; I really do. . . . If we didn't make [family] time, it—it would just be sad; it would be gone.

A medical or health regimen is the main reason for reordering time and scheduling. But do ill people stick to it? Maintaining the regimen derives from 1) defining the consequences of not keeping it, 2) learning to assess what one can do, 3) discerning immediate negative effects, 4) feeling life is under control, and 5) building accountability into the schedule.

If abandoning their regimen causes ill people to have immediate negative consequences, they are likely to keep it. For example, a woman with diabetes found herself in an emergency room after one failure to schedule her exercise and insulin in synchrony with her food intake. She said, "I got careless, a little sloppy and I could have died. I know I have to be more careful now." Similarly, if people believe their schedules help them keep illness contained, then they are inclined to continue them.

Fear of rapid deterioration or death prods certain ill people to keep a scheduled regimen. This fear looms largest just after a life-threatening crisis. A man with insulin-dependent diabetes explained, "My body hadn't let me down before and now it wanted to kill me. So I felt like I had a very powerful enemy very close to home. I was religious in my observance of my diet, making sure that I got exercise and ate at the right time right from the start. Well, I haven't kept it up like that but at first I was very absolute about it and I'd cut out alcohol altogether."

Like this man, ill people often maintain rigid regimens after a crisis, only to loosen or abandon them later. If they do not experience notable gains from their new routines, or do not notice encroaching symptoms when they begin to slip, then they are likely to drop schedules founded on illness. After staring at death during a crisis, ill people, not infrequently, distance themselves from it later. Hence, after surgery, heart patients maintain their exercise programs for several months but then let them lapse. A man with a heart condition said, "The doctor told me that I should be walking at least two miles a day. I started to but then with our busy season [at work], I've let it slip—what with overtime and all the stress."

A feeling that life is under control because of a schedule or regimen provides an incentive for keeping it. This feeling usually develops *after* people have reordered time and maintained their schedules. Following the schedule helps them minimize uncertainty; they believe that they are doing what they can to protect themselves and to preserve their lives (cf. Comaroff and Maguire 1981). These people traded putting effort into their schedules for gaining that sense of control. Why then do schedules become problematic?

Work and relationship tensions elicit feelings that life is out of control. A man with diabetes reflected, "I think that I smoke, eat the candy bar, or stop exercising when I feel like things are out of control. When life seems out of control, then I lose control [of his scheduled regimen]." A woman feared that she might lose her job. As she tried harder to please her supervisor, virtually all her time went to her work. She did not get sufficient rest or follow her diet. As she gained control over her livelihood, she felt that she lost more control over her health.

Building accountable routines into the schedule may help. But how does accountability work? To whom should ill people be accountable? And accountable from whose perspective?

Gaining acknowledgment of ill people's special needs and

their efforts to meet them without demeaning monitoring seems to work. A woman with multiple sclerosis took water exercise classes at the local swim club where she was part of a congenial group. Friends noted her presence or absence and commented sympathetically on it. Treating her exercise program as an important part of her social life encouraged her to continue it. Before, she found that she easily let exercise slide after several months.

The camaraderie, competition, and regular exercise in a cardiac rehabilitation treatment program also offer incentives for continuing to follow it. An accountability emerges that provides people with social support and rewards them for their efforts. Making the regimen part of a daily schedule helps people maintain it—if they work well with schedules and will plan, organize, and follow through. Some people regard streamlining their days as an engrossing puzzle to solve by making all the pieces of the puzzle fit smoothly. A number of people echoed this man's statement: "I have more time for important things because I schedule them now; I am more organized."

Accountability through sociability results from others caring—caring about these ill people and their progress or plight. Rather than separating ill people, scheduling here brings them into interaction with supportive others. In short, systematic support sustains the schedule (cf. Pearlin and Aneshensel 1986).

Accountability to self and to people other than spouse or caregiver widens the circle of concern. Ill people with a wider circle probably manage better than their counterparts who see themselves as only accountable to spouse, parent, or adult child. Being accountable only to the spouse about eating regularly, following diets, taking medications, pacing, and so on can make adversaries of the ill person and spouse, as lay practitioner and patient or as parent and child. Then the caregiver monitors and the patient sneaks. A diabetic sneaks drinks and junk food. A heart patient slips away for an ice cream cone instead of the prescribed walk. The adversary relation can grow, like an untreated wart. One woman had an "ornery" elderly uncle who had diabetes. She discovered that he had enlisted his former drinking buddies to bring him liquor in diet soda bottles. In addition, the neighbors supplied him with doughnuts and cookies. The competition between adversaries can deflect attention away from the reasons for the regimen as they become enmeshed in their competition for control.

Regimens and schedules change. Some people improve—markedly. They have a remission, benefit from a procedure, or complete their treatment successfully. Thus, ill people change schedules not only by extending, adapting, or revising them, but also through loosening, abandoning or reducing earlier schedules.

Loosening a schedule opens time slots and frees blocks of time. A remission of illness yields new hours of healthy time; the person feels alert, comfortable, and energetic. When Patricia Kennedy was in remission, she said, "It doesn't take me as long to shower, get dressed, fix meals and I don't need to exercise or rest as much. I have all this time now so what am I going to do with it?"

Nine years ago, Mark Reinertsen had a packed schedule of school, work, student teaching, community action groups, and psychological growth workshops—besides exhausting dialysis treatments three times a week. Then he received his second kidney transplant. He slowed down. Not simply because he could jettsion a huge chunk of his schedule. Not merely because the drugs for preventing transplant rejection ate his bones. But, because, in his words, "I'm not as concerned with getting everything into the day as I was. I've got a lot of free time this semester, too. I chose that. . . . When I was on dialysis, it was really to the point in my life where I didn't think I'd live past thirty, so I was trying to get everything in. And now I've got three months to go, I figure I'll make it, and there's a good chance of it. I'm not worried about getting it all in now."

Lenor Madruga had cancer, which resulted in losing her leg and part of her hip. After being fitted for a prothesis, she writes:

The routine daily functions that I had to do became easier and easier. Wearing my prothesis and going up and down the stairs became less of an effort. Doing the household chores only took half a day instead of the entire day. Cooking was so much quicker and less tiring on two legs rather than on one. At last, I was able to carry things to and from the table without having to dangle dishes and cups from hands which were already occupied with crutches. (1979:169)

More commonly, people I interviewed loosened their schedules because they could not manage them as their conditions worsened, as occurred with Mark Reinertsen some years later. They gave up work, leisure, and friends. These people loosened their schedules to allow for rest, regimen, symptoms, and crises. They intentionally slowed down. And by doing so, they could then better manage day-to-day fluctuations in their physical capabilities.

Perhaps the most difficult changes turn on abandoning a valued schedule and facing an unpredictable life. Most try to make the best of it by managing in whatever ways they can. Nancy Swenson described her schedule while she raised her children:

So I always had this struggle of working two jobs to maintain and support my kids and a lot of times to support my spouse and keep things going . . . I used to *push* myself. I worked a full-time job; I commuted to work [fifty-five miles away] and worked weekends at Western House [a bar and restaurant] when my children were younger, hand-milked two cows, bottle-fed calves, raised calves; we had chickens, raised my family, and now I am lucky if I can make it to the barn to feed the horses.

Like others who had diseases of unknown etiology, Nancy Swenson believed that her illness resulted from the strains of her prior life; she worked at relinquishing schedules. She remarked: "I am slowing down; I am enjoying people a lot more, the trees." She added, "I have a real phobia about schedules, a real phobia. It's like I enjoy going to church, but it can't be a schedule. It can't be that I have to be there every Sunday at 8:00, or I won't go. I don't know, it's like somebody says— hands me a schedule, oh, it's like freak city, I don't want any part of a schedule."

Giving up a full schedule can jolt anyone, particularly when it happens quickly. Workers quit jobs or are fired. Retirees cannot return to their prestigious volunteer positions. People who feel spent, however, initially relinquish their prior schedules with more relief than remorse, even when financial problems and loneliness result from leaving work. For some people, such as kidney dialysis patients, the rhythms of treatment formed a schedule. Many others structured their days by how they felt.

For a number of homebound people, activities beyond treatment and self-care routines became discomforting symbols of what they no longer could do and could no longer control. Unpredictable bad days disallow even following a reduced schedule. Several people dwelt on the anxiety they felt about getting to and getting through an anticipated event—Christmas dinner, a grand-daughter's wedding, a club's annual outing. May Morganson made plans to go to a special show at the art museum with a group of friends. Tickets were limited. Her friends had rented a bus and had made reservations for dinner afterwards. She worried for six weeks about being well enough to go.

Scheduled events also serve as symbols to other people, who note and comment upon whether the ill person attends. And like May Morganson, ill people look forward to the event for months or weeks ahead of time, only to feel desolate if they cannot attend it. Thus, they resisted scheduling because, as Nancy Swenson said, "scheduling leads to expectation and expectation leads to disappointment." Ann Rorty explained, "I try not to have too much [scheduled]—like tomorrow, I'm going to do this and this. I try not to set myself goals that I ought to reach; I try to be realistic about myself—what I can do and what I can't. If I can't do something that maybe I'd planned on—not to be too disappointed."

Juggling and Pacing

Making trade-offs depends upon juggling and pacing. In turn, effective juggling and pacing make life manageable. What do juggling and pacing mean in the lives of chronically ill people? When do they do it? How do they do it?

When people juggle, they balance activities with priorities, and that leads, in turn, to reorganizing and rescheduling events and tasks. As they think about pacing, they try to control the rate of movement during activities. Maintaining a job usually calls for intricate juggling and pacing.

Juggling and pacing become equivalent to managing daily life for many seriously ill people. Earlier high levels of activity and productivity lead to overestimating present capacity. Hence, learning to juggle and pace proceeds through trial and error— frustrating errors. Maureen Murphy disclosed, "My biggest thing that I've had to learn is to pace myself. 'Cause like when I feel really good, then I'll say, 'Oh, wow, I'm going to do everything. I am going to clean things from top to stern, you know, and I am going to make yeast bread and I'm going to do this and I'm going to do that.' And then you get halfway in the middle of it and all of a sudden, [groans] you're really wiped out."

The costs of overestimating capacity can be paid in embarrassment or pain. As Tina Reidel noted, "I have to be very careful to pace myself to get enough rest or else I may not be able to get up the next day. If I get too tired and take my muscles into fatigue, I get spasms. They're painful because they put all this stress on my joints, you know. If I'm not careful, I'll set myself back."

Frequently, incentives to keep on juggling and pacing result from responsibilities for others. A single mother commented, "I have to pace myself, not just for me, but for them [her two children]. Their father does very little for them. I doubt, and I think they do too, whether he would take them if I had a crisis." Other single mothers also foresaw no possibility of help from former husbands who had disappeared, become alcoholics, landed in jail, or who had simply married someone the children did not like.

The extent to which someone juggles and paces depends upon the possible trade-offs, available alternatives, and the degree of control he or she has over them. While a graduate student, Mark Reinertsen wrote his papers at the typewriter because he felt that he could not put the time and energy into revising. Lara Cobert dealt with her son's school problems and her developing symptoms one week and let her house go until the next. Nancy Swenson explained the kind of trade-off she considered with pacing: "If I stay up to 11:00, I know that I'll feel it the next day. It gives you pause when you think about making plans. I used to be the sort of person who would go in a minute. I can't maintain that pace. I ask myself now, 'Is it worth it?' I may decide to go, but I think about what it will cost me the next day, or even a couple of days."

If ill people can reorganize and control their schedules, shift burdens when needed, and adapt their pace, then juggling and pacing work well. For example, a retired woman decreed that her kidney dialysis treatments could not interfere with her aquatic exercise group, which had met regularly for over four years. She planned her treatments around her exercise group. Her husband took over cooking and housework on the days she had dialysis or needed more rest.

Juggling and pacing do not work when people have unlimited demands upon them but possess limited strength and endurance. A woman tried to juggle all the demands of her job and to pace herself so that she could get the most important and visible tasks completed, despite her frequent absences and slowed pace. But she was always behind, always trying to catch up. She would handle one major assignment and let others slide. Then she would have to work all weekend to try to catch up before the other undone tasks became visible. And if she worked all weekend, she had trouble getting through the next week. Another acute illness, another absence. If she rested all weekend, then she faced having panicky feelings about piles of work, discovery by co-workers, and another demeaning reprimand from her supervisor.

Many ill people juggle and pace to keep up with others who do not have the added burdens of illness and regimen. Paradoxically, some of these people discover that their juggling and pacing make it possible for them to outshine their peers. Their efforts take them beyond the worlds and the achievements of their peers. Consider the statement Vera Mueller made after she had returned to college for her B.A. degree:

Sam [her boyfriend] is so jealous of what I am doing; he's so jealous of my involvement with school. I have not had time for him to—swim around in his own confusion. . . . What I have had to do is withdraw from him. I have had to pull back my involvement because in order to be involved with him I have to work on his timeframe and he is mellow yellow and I'm not. And in the process we have lost a lot of what linked us together.

When people work, the juggling and pacing that they do to maintain their independence results in limiting, or even losing, friendships. Maintaining independence may even be an explicit trade-off for losing friends. When Sara Shaw was establishing her career, she observed, "I'm not—I don't know if reciprocal is the right word or not—I don't give 120 percent for my friends, I really don't. . . . Making a living is more important to me than anybody."

Then friends get jettisoned. Sara Shaw needed to pace her meals and rest periods, which occasionally resulted in disputes with friends. After waiting for a tardy friend with whom she had had dinner plans, she left. She reflected:

Well, I say what I need. I say it very bluntly a lot of times. . . . When I was talking with to Suzanne [the friend she had expected to meet] she was saying, "Well, I can see your point and I can see your justifications, you know, for things, but I don't feel like you can see mine at all." . . . I only trust myself, ultimately and stuff, and I *know* that if I don't eat or if I'm late [in eating], I know that I'm not going to be all right—that I have to do that. And so I'm real selfish in that kind of stuff. It's like I can see what she's saying, but I think that I overrule it. . . . If she can't be there, or, you know, they can't do it the way I need it, then too bad. And it's hard to have friends that way.

Juggling and pacing allow people to remain active, to maintain valued pursuits, to contain illness. They are able to preserve chunks of their earlier lives and previous selves. They keep pace with others and meet the terms set forth by others, be they employers, co-workers, or relatives. If illness remains in the background of their lives, ill people describe juggling and pacing as resulting from other concerns than symptoms and regimens—work, spouse's job, children's activities, family crises and the like. When a middle-aged woman suddenly experienced disturbing and disabling symptoms, she slowed down—markedly. Despite this change, she viewed her problems in juggling and pacing as derived from her newly retired husband's increased demands on her time and her son's drug use.

Lessons about juggling and pacing learned when very ill can last. These lessons take feelings into account as well as physical status. Sara Shaw had an opportunity to get a prestigeous job. She said, "Most people would jump for it no matter what, but I'm not ready for it and I know that; I learned to follow my own pacing when I was sick." She added, "Emotionally, I'll be making jumps that I won't let myself do for a long time, a lot longer. I don't jump emotionally. I don't see myself leave anything like that [her steady job] at the drop of a hat for a long time. I'd say my emotions go first, then I watch it and try it out for a long time before I make any moves."

Organizing, simplifying, reordering time, juggling, and pacing also become a part of caregiving. Whether or not caregiving can continue rests, in large part, on effective control of these processes, particularly when the bulk of the work falls on one caregiver.

Juggling and pacing get complicated when both "patient" and "caregiver" have chronic illnesses. But even if reciprocity in juggling has existed for years, one partner's more rapid decline, more visible disability, or more serious diagnosis shifts the balance. That partner becomes defined as the patient and the other as caregiver. When this definition rules the household, some "patients" will not budge from their "appointed" roles, almost as if they have received tenure as patients.

Subsequently, the needs of the caregiver seem miniscule, or nonexistent. If so, then an ill caregiver struggles with his or her illness almost entirely alone. An older man was steeped in self-pity about developing severe heart disease shortly after his retirement. He expected his wife to attend to his fears, symptoms, and routines. Two years later, she had a mastectomy, followed by radiation and chemotherapy. Though these procedures might shift the patient-caregiver roles, in this case they did not. He still expected her to juggle her needs around his. Here, long-established patterns gave precedence to his needs.

When someone claims tenure as the patient, virtually all the juggling and pacing falls on the caregiver. This arrangement might work if the caregiver's physical and psychological health holds out. But often it doesn't: the relationship deteriorates; home health services become prohibitive or undependable; the caregiver dies.

Yet when partners have long taken both of their needs into account, they exchange patient and caregiver roles as needed for years. Despite having had four heart attacks, an older man took interest in his wife's pursuits—he drove her on errands when she was tired, typed her college papers for her, involved himself in the household and family activities. She had cared for him during his heart attacks; he cared for her after she had a stroke. These reciprocities buffered the strains of caregiving and gave the couple a sense of completion of the relationship.

As ill people remake their lives through planning, organizing, and making trade-offs, they learn what it means to live with illness and disability. Tiny daily tasks such as getting bathed and dressed, cooking, and driving reveal images of an emerging self. For many, the learning continues as their conditions and treatments change, for the better as well as for the worse. For others, learning to reconstruct their lives in new or different ways simply is not possible. Instead, they jettison the tasks or depend on somebody else to do them. Withdrawal and lowered expectations follow. But those who invent ways to handle those tasks that pose major barriers and make trade-offs to preserve valued pursuits often gain a sense of accomplishment and pride.

Illness, the Self, and Time

In this section, I turn directly to relationships between illness, the self, and time. The elusive experience of lived time takes on sharper form when studied from the vantage point of what ill people think, do, and feel about time. People with chronic illnesses provide mirrors of time and self for other adults, because time and even having a self become so problematic for them. Hence, their thoughts, feelings, and actions about time reflect a distilled version of adult life.

In Chapter 7, I address how ill people structure and restructure the present. To do so, I look closely at the mundane ways that people try to structure time, and at their ordinary language that shapes meanings of their attempts to do so. I emphasize what the present looks and feels like when illness has made life uncertain. I show how time perspectives reflect the ways that people structure time. Chronic illness can drastically affect what people believe that they can and should do in the present. Hence, their ways of structuring the present are likely to shift as their health changes. For many people, changing their ways of structuring time also means changing their perspectives on past, present, and future—which is often a much harder task. But should they do so, maintaining the restructured time becomes habit.

Ideas about the past influence the present and future. In Chapter 8, I discuss how people take note of their past with illness. They create bench marks and illness chronologies of this past. They attribute meanings of some bench marks for their developing selves. They define certain events as turning points. They find some events so significant that their effects shape feelings and self-images for months or years. I show how past feeling-laden events become turning points for self, not simply of illness.

From there I move to Chapter 9, the last major chapter of the book. In it I propose that people's self-concepts come to be tied to the past, present,

*or future. Time provides implicit ways of knowing and defining the self.
People come to treat the past, present, or future as pivotal for organizing
concepts of themselves although they usually remain unaware of how
rooted their self-concepts are in time. Lessons that ill people began to
learn by restructuring time and rethinking their ideas about it, if continued, have consequences for locating their self-concepts in time. Those
lessons may be forced upon ill people by growing disability and increased
loss of autonomy. A quasi-institutional living arrangement by itself
forces an individual to restructure time and promotes a revised time
perspective. Furthermore, the meanings of past marker events influence
feelings about and definitions of self that may keep people in the past. In
short, I argue that the social conditions of experiencing chronic illness
foster taken-for-granted ways of anchoring the self in the past, present,
or future.*

7

Time Perspectives and Time Structures

Living one day at a time. Yeah. That's what I tried to work on. . . . Every day was just a struggle. I'd take painkillers and that didn't work so it had to be every day. Every day it seemed like the arthritis was different . . . and it wouldn't go away. Sometimes it was just like really horrible and other times it was less. That's supposed to be one of the factors, this up and down. . . . I think since the arthritis has gone into remission it's not so much, you know, every day, but I still try to look at it as just every day is a new day.

Living one day at a time was living on the edge, the razor's edge. But I think when I was taking one day at a time was really frightening because each day would be so different. And then it would be a big struggle just to get to work, just to get dressed, just to get to the bus. I would just concentrate on the one day.

Living one day at a time. Being on the edge. Searching for relief from pain. For three years, Tina Reidel had had unremitting pain from active rheumatoid arthritis. Time shrank into the present except when drowned by waves of fear. "Will it always be like this? Will it never go away?" At those points, her image of the future overwhelmed her.

During this period, Tina tried to get through the work week one day at a time. On Saturdays, she usually stayed in bed—spent and tormented by pain. On Sundays, friends offered her rides to the meetings of her Eastern spiritual group. Unable to fulfill others' expectations, she felt their irritations, disappointments, and accusations. Her lover expected her to do the housecleaning; it remained undone. Her supervisor demanded

169

that she finish typing his reports; she seldom made his deadlines. Co-workers urged her to go on disability, and her supervisor bullied her. However, she felt that she could keep the job by taking one day at a time.

Later, Tina Reidel's arthritis improved for a few months. Her pain markedly lessened and her fears subsided. She began to look toward a future. As her time perspective began to expand to include the future, her social worlds widened. New questions arose: "Why am I in this relationship?" "Where am I going?" New possibilities emerged; a fellow spiritual seeker asked her to marry him. Tina began to explore maps of the future.

How does experiencing chronic illness affect time perspective? Conversely, how does time perspective affect experience? Under which conditions does someone's time perspective shift and change? What views do people have of the present? How do they use it? How might their experience of the present shape their perspectives of past and future?

As evident in the preceding chapters, serious chronic illness forces active men and women to restructure time. In turn, changes in structuring time promote changes in perspectives about time. For clarity, a *time structure* denotes how people frame, organize, and use time. Consistent with Barley (1988), beginnings, endings, rhythms, cycles, and changes all contribute to a time structure. In contrast, a *time perspective* means ideas, beliefs, and views about the content, structure, and experience of time.

In this chapter, I look at the present and examine how ill people's thoughts, feelings, and actions toward it shape their time structure and reshape their time perspective. Meanings of the present set time horizons and give substance to images of past and future (Jaques 1982; Mead 1932). Ill people develop prescriptions and implicit goals for relating to the present, such as living one day at a time or recapturing the past. Throughout, I explicate their implicit meanings about time and outline conditions that prompt them to revise, adapt, or change a current time perspective, or encourage them to resume an earlier one.

Altered Time Structures and Shifting Time Perspectives

Forced changes in structuring time can cause shifts in time perspective.[1] When does time structure shape time perspective? What contributes to retaining or maintaining an earlier time perspective? When are time structures and time perspectives incongruent?

Temporal Incongruence

Temporal incongruence develops when time perspectives are incompatible and inconsistent with time structures. When health has noticeably declined, a previous time structure based on multiple time commitments seldom works anymore. Yet ill people's assumptions about viewing and using time may not fit the time structures that their bodies permit. Following his near-death crisis, a middle-aged man said, "My time perspective has been jilted around a little bit." Alternatively, immersion in a lengthy episode can lead to adopting the time structure and perspective of convalescence unwittingly. Should these people return to earlier pursuits, they may find that their assumptions about viewing and structuring time are incongruent with those of other people.

Temporal incongruence tends to be discovered through daily events. A woman with arthritis took a full-time job. She had difficulty getting enough rest, doing her water exercises, keeping the house, and spending time with her husband. When her daughter returned to the area, she added socializing and occasional babysitting to her already packed schedule. Another flare-up decimated her schedule. She said, "That last flare-up made it clear to me that being that busy is just not that important—it's too much for me, but it is hard to change the way I think about using time."

Such realizations do, however, prompt shifts in time perspective. In turn, when an ill person's shifting time perspective butts against that of other people's, conflict results. Conflicting time perspectives are played out in daily plans, priorities, and pursuits, as people structure time. However, underlying assumptions about time typically remain hidden. Instead, people make mutual accusations of blame, poor motivation, power-grabbing, and the like.

Temporal incongruence results when intimates do not share similar ways of thinking about and structuring time. Hence, conflict emerges when making daily schedules and projecting timetables (Roth 1963; Zerubavel 1981). A middle-aged man had convalesced for several months when his wife began to push him to go back to work. He remarked:

> My wife put it to me one day; she said, in one of her less charitable moments . . . "What are you going to do? What are you going to do today? Well, what are you going to do today? *Recover?*" And I went and I thought, I said, "What I'm going to do today is try to live my life without reacting to structures that I can't meet [or] cope with anyway. And that's basically the whole philosophy of life I guess I am approaching the world with these days. At least to the extent that I can. And it's really severely important to me—to not live my life according to somebody else's, or some external structures that I can't cope with.

This man found meaning in his illness by explicating problems that had existed before it. By devoting the present to search the past, one hopes to avoid recreating it in the future. Yet to a partner, the ill person's present timeout or extended convalescence foretells continued illness and a curtailed life. Thus, the partner prods the ill person to resume an earlier time perspective and structure. The process occurs in reverse when an ill man or woman adheres to an earlier time perspective and time structure but the partner believes it now inappropriate or impossible and argues for change (Speedling 1982).

Problems in structuring time may precede illness. Subsequently, illness causes an already shaky time structure to crumble. At the very least, illness illuminates and magnifies the rough spots that affect daily time structures, such as financial problems, marital conflict, and job instability. Dealing with these problems leads to shifts in time perspective.

An untenable time structure may derive from external demands upon the ill one. Time shortens because of the interruptions from other people. Children, co-workers, and demanding spouses all affect an ill person's time structure. Four years ago, Nancy Swenson's chaotic household wreaked havoc with her attempts to structure her time. Her foster daughter stole from her purse and lied at school. Her adult daughter separated from her husband and moved in and out. Then her son-in-law moved in briefly. Her dogs clamored for attention; her mother demanded it. Helpers occasionally came to work with her mother, but relied on Nancy for direction. During this period, Nancy suffered from insomnia. Fatigue, combined with other symptoms, impaired her mental concentration as well as her physical functioning.

The structure of Nancy Swenson's day resulted from the demands imposed by her mother's care and behavior. Her day shrank to uneven segments, interrupted minutes, and brief seconds when she could focus her attention. The chaotic household magnified and intensified Nancy's fatigue and difficulty in concentrating. Further, exacerbations of her illness directly affected her mother, whose disruptiveness then escalated. Nancy explained:

> But my mom can see and tell when I'm not feeling well. But with the Alzheimer's she knows something is wrong, but her brain doesn't tell her how to deal with it. . . . She gets angry at me and makes things very difficult for me. And I get to where I—I just don't even want her to be in the same house with me. . . . She just won't leave me alone. . . . And if I'm trying to get dinner ready and I'm already feeling bad, she's in front of the refrigerator. Then she goes to put her hand on the stove and I got the fire on. And then she's in front of the microwave and then she's in front of the silverware drawer. And—and if I send her out she gets mad at me. And then it's awful. That's when I have a really, a really bad time.

If Nancy tried to work on paying bills, her mother took her pen and scattered the bills. If she attempted to fill out Medi-Cal [Medicaid] forms, her mother hid her glasses. Though Nancy kept her time perspective close to the present, her present rapidly disappeared. Chaos devours time. Illness magnified Nancy's inability to manage time and to structure her life comfortably. She said, "I think, instead of just sitting here you could be doing paperwork. You could be getting all the doctor bills together and doing this and doing that. And I feel myself procrastinating. Well maybe tomorrow will be a better day. And the next thing I know, the time—time is gone."

Reorganization at work can make a manageable illness unmanageable as new time structures become untenable. Productivity speedups due to reorganization, promotion, or layoffs of co-workers wreck time structures. Several individuals had found it hard to handle their workload before a change increased it. Afterwards, they could not handle it. A corporate takeover had left a middle-aged salesman responsible for covering a larger area and for making higher profits in a tighter market. He felt that these changes contributed to his heart disease:

> I worked for Healthtech Pharmaceuticals and we sold blood therapeutic products. And I felt like I was a used car salesman at times, because everything was based on price and I would be running all around the countryside delivering vials of blood here and there and the other place, getting prices from the company, kind of fibbing to the company, telling them that my competition was lower so they would give me a lower price, you know. And, I was working out all kinds of deals. It was really traumatic.

Conversely, the tempo and time perspective imbedded in an ill person's social world can mask illness and affect mood but, simultaneously, provide an untenable time structure for maintaining his or her financial independence. For example, John Garston lived in a cluster of cabins where most of the residents led "Bohemian" lifestyles as artists, poets, and aging hippies. Distances between cabins were short and the pace and tempo of life was unhurried, so moving slowly was hardly noticeable. Further, several neighbors also had financial crises, little work, and were concerned with immediate needs like rent and food. A time structure with a slow tempo combined with a time perspective based in the immediate present can make taking initiative and giving extra effort especially difficult when one is ill. John's work in antique restoration largely depended upon his own resourcefulness in obtaining it and upon his perseverance in doing it. He said:

> I'm real lazy. That's contributed greatly to, you know, the illness and the laziness are just going—they're going back and forth contributing. . . . I just sit around and diddle around instead of—instead of doing, doing chores or doing this and that. . . . There have been periods when I have had very high energy, where I've worked twenty hours a day for, you know, a year at a time or so, and—or more, and had a lot of drive. And then, you know, something's happened to just blow things away.

John believed that his illness contributed to and magnified his current apathy and lassitude. His time perspective remained in the present yet his time structure led to experiencing time as moving swiftly. He shortened the day by starting it as late as possible (after his usual early morning insomnia), by ending it early, and by breaking it into segments. He commented: "The days pass amazingly swiftly for someone as bored as I am [laughs] . . . 'cause I sit and diddle around and read and drink coffee and smoke cigarettes, and all of a sudden it's—you know, and I—of course I try to go to bed as early as I can. Try to sleep as late as I can."

Role Models of Structuring Time

Lengthy treatment in a medical facility permits ill people to witness what happens to patients with similar conditions. As a result, some people resist letting illness take over their lives because they have visible, immediate, and negative role models of those who do. Simultaneously, they may find themselves becoming role models for others because they have lives beyond illness and treatment. When he was a graduate student, Mark Reinertsen mentioned, "It's like I'm the role model because I'm the only one actively doing something, at least on my shift. And it's like they all look up to me and I'm not sure that I want that. It's like a crazy responsibility and I'm not sure that I really want that."

Because Mark Reinertsen pursued interests beyond dialysis, the staff liked the way he structured time for them. His pursuits were noteworthy—exemplary. Consequently, the staff also expected him to be an exemplary dialysis patient. Mark said:

> The thing that bothers me is when I come to dialysis first of all, it's a free time for me; it's a time that I don't have anything scheduled that I have to do. I can do anything I want. I can read; I can watch a soap opera, which I do quite often; I can sleep. And that's four hours. And I bring what I want to eat, not necessarily what's on my diet, but what I want to eat. These are things that other people look at like, "how incorrigible," when you are definitely on a diet. I bring olives, potato chips, cheese dip. One nurse came up to me and said, "Alicia really looks up to you, what do you think she thinks about that diet?" It's like now I have to watch what I bring to eat there because I'm a role model there so it's a whole different role to be in.

More frequently, the staff choose patients as role models who fit both their interests and their regimens into their time structure. For example, an older woman was initially devastated by having kidney failure. But after she became acclimated to dialysis, she became the staff's annointed role model. She said:

> There's a lady up in Fairville who just started dialysis up there and the social worker wanted to know if I would talk to her and tell her that you can still have a life and be on dialysis. I'm going to . . . talk with her about the diet, your fears of all the other things and about dialysis. I'm going to tell her that you can schedule around it and still have a quality life.

Harry Bauer's diligence made him a role model for others in his cardiac rehabilitation program. Though long retired, he nevertheless maintained an active schedule that included rigorous exercise. He described a typical day: "Still get up at 4 o'clock." I asked, "Then what do you do?" He said:

Well I read; I read a lot of stuff in the stock market. Then at 5:30 my wife and I go over to our grandson's and she babysits over there, our grandson, and I come home usually about—it's around 8:00 and fix myself some breakfast, go for my—I'll either go for my three-mile walk first and then eat breakfast. I usually do it that-a-way, and then after breakfast, I'll ride five miles on my bike and then this afternoon, I'll do another five miles.

In contrast, negative role models structure time in ways that either preclude, ignore, or contradict regimens, or encourage wallowing in illness. Negative role models prod an ill person to maintain or create a time structure based on maintaining cherished involvements as well as physical and mental health. For example, Mark Reinertsen viewed a young woman whose anorexia had resulted in kidney failure as a negative role model. He observed that her life had shrunk to coming to dialysis and being a helpless victim. He remarked, "I don't want to listen to that. I don't want to be like that."

People who had active lives before try to create time structures that permit them to be active and productive while ill. But even active men and women eventually have to slow down. A new endeavor may reveal the changes in structuring time. In turn, the changed time structure prompts shifts in time perspectives. For example, except for timeouts for his transplant and acute illnesses, Mark Reinertsen had maintained a normal pace through his teaching credential program and practice teaching. But five years later, he could not handle the same pace as his peers in graduate school. The contrast in time structure was striking to him. His classmates, who held jobs, moved through the program on time; it took him 50 percent longer to complete it, despite taking a lighter load and devoting 100 percent of his time to it.

A highly structured professional training program provides clear indicators of timing and pacing. Set timemarkers denote beginnings and endings and chart whether one is ahead, behind, or on time. Due to an inheritance, Mark Reinertsen did not have to work after he graduated. Instead, he took a break to recoup from the rigors of graduate school and to enjoy his newfound affluence. That period became a "natural" break in his life, which he defined as a time for himself. However, he also suffered numerous complications at that time. But since he was taking a break, how he perceived and structured time—and how much time illness now took—remained less apparent than when he had deadlines, schedules, and cohorts with which to compare himself.

Living One Day at a Time

Living one day at a time means dealing with illness—each day—but only one at a time. When people do so, they hold future plans and even ordinary pursuits in abeyance. Their future is unsettled, or entirely uncertain. For most people, living one day at a time tacitly acknowledges their fragility.

Living one day at a time also allows people to focus on illness, treatment, and regimen without being overcome by dashed hopes and unmet expectations. Taking this stance provides guidelines for functioning each day and confers some sense of control. By concentrating on the present, ill people avoid or minimize thinking about further disability and death.

The felt need to live one day at a time can drastically alter one's time perspective. Living this way pulls the person's attention into the present and pushes once projected futures further away. Earlier visions of the future recede without disruption and slip away, perhaps almost unnoted. The present is compelling and, eventually, may seem rewarding. If so, the content of time changes; moments become longer and fuller.

Living one day at a time is a strategy for managing chronic illness and structuring time. Moreover, it also provides a way of managing self while facing uncertainty. It gives a sense of control over one's actions and, by extension, a sense of control over self and situation. Embracing this strategy also alters time perspective.

When ill people feel compelled to live one day at a time, they try to relinquish past visions of their future, despite their earlier commitment to those visions. A sixty-year-old woman with a minor heart condition cared for her husband who had serious heart disease. Because her mother and aunts had lived well into their nineties, she expected to live at least thirty more years and to survive her husband. He had lost his job, just three years before he could retire. While she anxiously attended to him, she planned to get a job for the first time in almost forty years. After a crucial house repair wiped out their life savings, she felt immense pressure to find work. Shortly thereafter, she suffered a small stroke from which she made a good initial recovery. She said, "I have to see it [her CVA] as a warning. I can't let myself get so anxious. I have to live one day at a time."

For this woman, changing her time perspective constituted a radical shift. Her time perspective changed from looking forward to an attenuated old age to living one day at a time. She had to work at it. Because her earlier time perspective had made the future real and vivid, the possibility of a foreshortened life shocked her. Although she had described herself as "nervous" and "high strung" long before her stroke, afterwards, she saw her anxiety as life-threatening. She said, "I just can't let myself get so upset. I can't try to do as much, and I have to keep calmer about what I do."

To her, living one day at a time meant monitoring her emotions about daily irritations and trying to control her fears about disability and death. It also meant reducing her daily schedule to decrease her panic about not getting everything done. Her emotional monitoring took precedence in structuring her days. She reduced her community work, household tasks, and family events, and deferred the job search. Her family also defined her CVA as a serious warning and encouraged her to live one day at a time.

Like others, this woman believed that she faced death and that her emotions could cause it. Such men and women feel coerced into living one day at a time. They force it upon themselves, almost with clenched teeth. Here, living one day at a time resembles learning an unfamiliar, disagreeable lesson in grammar school; it is an unwelcome prerequisite to staying alive.

At one point, Patricia Kennedy faced losing her physical independence again. For her, expressing fear helped her to look at her growing disability and brought her back to living one day at a time. Subsequently, she felt more control over her fear and her life. She said of her fear:

> I have to verbalize it. I usually cry. I've cried a lot in the last week. Sometimes, Kathy, I feel better after I have cried . . . because it is a venting of the fears. And the doctor—the neurologist the other day was telling me, "You know, if you come face to face with what you are afraid of and *look* at it, then you can deal with it." And I think that that's the truth because the bottom line was— when I first started getting it in my leg . . . I was scared to death that I would be in a wheelchair and that's the bottom line fear. The more recent fear is that if I go on the ACTH [steroid treatment] I will have to go into the hospital, and I don't want to do that. So I cried a lot about that last night. But then I think I've got to where I can take each day at a time.

For her, living one day at a time included relinquishing some future plans—retirement projects, private colleges for her sons, expensive vacations. For people who once had a future mapped out in detail, living one day at a time not only sweeps away their future time perspective, it overturns their time structure. Patricia Kennedy remarked:

> When you've been a person who set long-term goals, then short-term goals are hard. And not being able to make a commitment is really difficult. I was saying to someone just the other day, "Not being able to say, 'Oh, I can drive or I can do that, go to that function in two weeks,' because I don't know—that's hard for me."

Living one day at a time reveals emotions embedded in the experience of illness. Many ill people, especially older people, express greater fear of dependence, debility, and abandonment than of death. Living one day at a time helps to reduce their fear that the future will be worse than the present. During a series of setbacks, Mark Reinertsen murmured, "I try to live one day at a time because it is just less frightening." Later, he observed, "I could just get really tied up in what might happen [death or further deterioration], since so much has happened in the last six months [multiple complications and iatrogenic diseases]. But what good does it do? I can only handle today."

Similarly, Kathleen Lewis writes about learning to live one day at a time after her diagnosis of lupus erythematosus:

> I found myself consumed with fear of what the future would hold and longing to have things back the way they were in the past.
>
> Shadows of my new life began emerging, but I found myself imprisoned by the bars of yesterday and tomorrow. In a mere survival struggle I found myself praying, "Give me this day my daily bread," trying desperately to focus on one day at a time—one moment at a time.
>
> I found that it took intentional effort not to dwell on thoughts from the past and future, but to concentrate on my todays. Taking one moment, one day at a time was more manageable. It set me free to enjoy and experience where I was.
>
> I would slip back into my old patterns and have to will myself back to the day-to-day, moment-by-moment frame of mind. I realized that I couldn't control what thoughts came into my head, but I could control what I did with them. (1985:25–26)

Living one day at a time mutes "negative" emotions—fear, guilt, anger, and self-pity—and even gives one a sense of control over them.[2] By living one day at a time, Mark Reinertsen said that he didn't punish himself for not following his strict diet earlier. A woman said that it lessened her regrets about forced retirement. Another woman found it helped her to check her anger and to limit those nagging "why me?" questions. She remarked, "I don't keep prying into the past; I've quit that and I can let it go."

Further, living one day at a time quiets feelings of being overwhelmed by illness and regimen. By exerting control over the day, people avoid feeling that managing illness is an unbearable life sentence. A woman with diabetes remarked, "If I kept thinking that I can never have chocolate or cookies again, then I'd feel overwhelmed and deprived. But if I just think, 'I'm not going to have any chocolate or cookies today—period,' then I feel all right about it."

By gaining a feeling of control over the day, ill people believe that they have made some improvement and are winning their struggle against illness. Before severe heart disease forced his retirement, Harry Bauer's fast-paced position meant weighty responsibilities. Ten years later, he said, "I kind of take it [life] from day to day. Even though my investing's on the long term, I don't, uhm, really see that I'd make much changes in the future, probably go along like I am doing . . . nothing bothers me anymore. . . . I used to worry about things. I don't worry about nothing anymore. It flows off my back like water off a duck's back."

Living one day at a time helped Harry Bauer reduce his fear and structure his day. Moreover, he gained control over his life. Paradoxically, by gaining a sense of control, he again foresaw having a future. He said, "I feel great since the surgery; I feel better with the exercise program and diet than I have in years. I'm planning on living another twenty years!"

Through either present intent or prior life structure, living one day at a time can become a habit. An elderly woman cared for her invalid husband. Her health failed as she aged and as he deteriorated. She had, in many ways, lived one day at a time for much of her life. Their lack of plans did not bother her nearly as much as her arduous days and her husband's ungratefulness and refusal to acknowledge her health problems. The doctor first estimated that she would have to care for him for only two years. It stretched into seven. She had been living one day at a time for so long that it had become habitual. Their situation also continued the time perspective and structure of their earlier years during which they had only painted a future in broad strokes rather than in fine detail.

Certainly, living one day at a time can serve as a strategy for handling relationships, in addition to coping with illness. Further, living one day at a time can indicate the fluid, uncertain future. Her own illness, limited finances, and the job of caring for her mother with Alzheimer's, led Nancy Swenson to live one day at a time. Also, she said about having Kerry, her foster daughter:

> It's temporary. I'm taking that one day at a time. A lot's going to depend on Kerry and a lot of it is a lot to ask of an eleven year old

because, you know, especially the environment she has been through [many moves, no father, a mother on drugs]. But like I've told Kerry, I can't have hassles in my life. My life is too short. I don't know how much time I've got.

Living one day at a time means giving full attention to the present. Yet it is hard to do. And living one day at a time applies to other problems besides illness. Hence, living one day at a time can take varied forms. Ill people may: 1) attend to it in parts of their lives, but project a future in others, 2) concentrate on living one day at a time during hard times, such as turning points, or 3) begin to live one day at a time as a permanent accommodation to illness or to life.

Like many elders, an old woman lived one day at a time but also framed a tentative future. She concentrated on her rest, daily routine, and regimen. Her most demanding tasks were meal preparation and walking the distance of one block to her mailbox. Her regimen involved stretching her joints each morning so that she could cook and walk, counting out her medications, and taking them at the correct intervals. She projected a future no more than six months ahead, which coincided with her niece's visit. Otherwise, she did not chart a future.

While in crises, many ill people live one day at a time as a temporary strategy. They also do so when they wait for suspected bad news. Living one day at a time is a way to shift down and concentrate on immediate hurdles. Subsequently, ill people restructure time. They renegotiate or relinquish earlier commitments. They narrow their territory and reduce their activities. They stop driving, avoid outings, add rest periods to their day. They step up their monitoring. They do all this willingly—if it has worked in the past to stave off a full-blown episode or to avoid a particularly nasty treatment.

People may adopt living one day at a time reluctantly as a temporary strategy for getting through a hard time, like following a crash diet for a period but expecting a later release to freedom. In the meantime, living one day at a time may provide them with a protective shield against an onslaught of troubles.[3]

A crisis certainly can renew awareness of death. For some, living one day at a time after a crisis may provide a way to find more meaning in life. By focusing closely on priorities, ill people begin to define their values. As one man said:

> I'm relating to time differently in other ways [beyond scheduling], I think more subtle and more deep ways. . . . We all know that we are going to die. We all know that we're just here temporarily, but we all try, nevertheless, to avoid that fact. . . . And to that sense, I think there's been a change because at least I'm actively trying to keep that in my attention . . . because I think it is a lot healthier to live with that idea constantly in your mind that every breath could be your last one. . . . So that adjusts things about what is important to you.

A life-threatening crisis, however, does not necessarily lead to living one day at a time. If people have always looked to future horizons, they do not easily shorten their sights to the present and make living one day at a time a permanent strategy. Mike Reilly saw himself as a future-driven, competitive "Type A" man. He said of living one day at a time:

> I think it's self-defeating. Good Christians could ask me for their daily bread or something like that but no, I want more than that. And I haven't lost that and that's part of my—call it anger or rage or frustration or something. . . . I can't accept one day at a time—I just—I've tried it and it worked then [in the aftermath of crisis], but as I'm getting healthy now, I don't want to pursue that.

Living one day at a time remains an onerous strategy for many people. The future seeps into the present or the past floods it. If illness subsides, these people allow images of the future to reflect upon their present. When that occurs, living one day at a time will no longer be necessary, because these people now have hope of once again seeing a future.

The social setting and involvements of an ill person can foster living one day at a time. For example, a few very old people in a board and care home still possessed their mental faculties. They had a tacit agreement to refrain from discussing their future prospects. By doing so, they coped with a living arrangement that disturbed and distressed them.

Living one day at a time can spur someone to find meaning and fulfillment. It can become a path to celebrating life rather than only a forced strategy for sustaining it (Lewis 1985). Fear of death melts away. As Nancy Swenson reflected:

> I'm not afraid to die at all. I would just like to have things in order before I die, but I'm not afraid to die. And I hope that it's quickly and that I don't suffer. . . . Even if I had to go to a home, I think I could even make the best of a home. . . . I feel I've lived a pretty full life, am pretty interesting. I could probably write a book, and it would probably be interesting enough to read. And what more could I ask for?

Existing from Day to Day

Existing from day to day occurs when a person plummets into continued crises that rip life apart. It reflects loss of control of health and the wherewithal to keep life together.

Existing from day to day means constant struggle for daily survival. Poverty and lack of support contribute to and complicate that struggle. Hence, poor and isolated people usually plummet further and faster than affluent individuals with concerned families. Loss of control extends to being unable to obtain necessities—food, shelter, heat, medical care.

The struggle to exist keeps people in the present, especially if they have continual problems in getting the basic necessities that middle-class adults take for granted. Yet other problems can assume much greater significance for these people than their illness—a violent husband, a runaway child, an alcoholic spouse, the overdue rent.

Living one day at a time differs from existing from day to day. Living one day at a time provides a strategy for controlling emotions, managing life, dimming the future, and getting through a troublesome period. It involves managing stress, illness, or regimen, and dealing with these things each day to control them as best as one can. It means concentrating on the here and now and relinquishing other goals, pursuits, and obligations.

In contrast, existing from day to day means getting through

the day, scraping by; life is beyond control. Poverty and crises can preclude attending to health. Constant crises with no viable solutions, no resolutions, can overwhelm anyone. A man with diabetes has a few drinks to calm down. A woman with a heart condition abandons her exercise program when her son gets enmeshed in the juvenile justice system. An impoverished elderly woman tries to stretch her medication by taking only half of the dosage.

May Morganson's retirement income barely covered her rent. Soon she could not afford her strict diet. She relied on her tiny garden and food her neighbors occasionally brought. As her condition worsened, she could not stand or sit without pain. She could not garden or cook, so she stretched a few convenience foods and accepted sporadic help from her neighbors.

Loss of control can raise questions about whether ill people will live and whether they want to. Their time perspective shortens as they struggle through each day. When Mark Reinertsen had multiple complications from renal failure and a series of acute illnesses, he observed, "I'm living on the edge—I'm just going from day to day, hoping I don't fall off." A woman said, "I am so sick that it takes everything I've got just to keep going today."

For a woman with terminal emphysema, existing from day to day involved regimens, apparatus, and getting needed assistance so that she could live to see another day. She could not use her expensive medication and apparatus if she had no one to help her. Without assistance, she had to exist from day to day. John Garston's emphysema was less advanced. His condition contributed to his plight but did not wholly structure it. For him, existing from day to day involved having food and shelter. He disclosed, "My thoughts are just totally from day to day." John's emphysema curtailed his pursuits and his poverty curtailed his attending to his emphysema. He described existing from day to day:

I'm literally concerned about say, my next meal, my current shelter, and things like that. And being concerned about all that, solely concerned about that doesn't help me, in fact it hurts me in a lot of ways because I'm not able to do long-range thinking. A person that doesn't have to worry about living day to day can be more concerned with long-range health plans.

John Garston received no help except from a few friends. But even those who have help from family and social programs may be forced into existing from day to day. Maria Goodvage (1988) presents Bill's story of his environmental illness. By his mid-forties, Bill had to abandon a professional career because the chemicals in urban settings made him sick. His mother and sister paid for treatment, equipment, and a cabin. He had received Supplemental Security Income of which almost two-thirds went to prescriptions; the remainder covered food and payments to his mother for upkeep on the cabin. Later, when his mother could not handle the expenses, Bill eliminated most of his prescriptions in order to pay for the cabin. Goodvage writes:

> He can't make ends meet. Pacific Gas & Electric is about to shut off his electricity if he doesn't pay the $541 he owes for five months of service. He's in debt to a pharmacy for $450.
>
> Since Bill cut back on his medication, his IQ has gone from 140 to 85, according to research neuropsychiatrist Shiela Bastien of Berkeley. "It's really sad to see a man with such brilliance and creativity slip into a state over which he has no control."
>
> Now he speaks with a stutter he shed years ago. Headaches and dizziness keep him in bed for days at a time. (1988:15)

Prior expectations of being able to control one's life make existing from day to day unbearable. A relentless slide into poverty intensifies anger and panic. Middle-class and professional people can find themselves so poor and debilitated that they cannot function. Their fates both amaze and daze them.

What is a day like when people exist from day to day? How do they spend the day? During a "good" day, they fill time. During a "bad" day, they experience chaos. When people "fill" time, the day has large blocks of time, which haunt them. Filling time seldom involves structured activity. It means struggling to rest, worrying, watching television, perhaps, reading, but most likely, simply trying to exist (Calkins 1970). Contrasts between the present and the past make filling time apparent. John Garston said:

> I just go from day to day so—I don't have the long-term worries [about his health]. . . . I'm just existing from day to day, yeah, yeah. . . . Filling up the time. . . . I don't go to bed satisfied. You know, I go to bed because the day is over. . . . [A few years before] I had done interesting things and I had hope of more interesting things on the morrow. . . . Being interested in something like this [antique restoration] . . . encompasses a lot more than a job.

Filling time occurs while someone waits for resolution—to improve, to die, to get help. John Garston existed from day to day as he waited for resolution of his court case. He admitted that "I have a lot of stress on me right now. I have this crazy court thing, and everything, that's driving me nuts. My oldest friend, who's my attorney, he just had emergency heart surgery and had to drop out and things like that, the trouble with my child and everything—on top of nagging poverty [laughs]."

Constant crises. No resolution in sight. Spiraling problems and devastating illness. Chaos. John Garston's illness was intrusive, but not wholly debilitating. Nancy Swenson, in contrast, sometimes felt barely alive. In addition, she felt overwhelmed by her other daily problems. Conditions at home worsened as her mother became incontinent and more volatile. When Nancy's illness flared up again, she said, "I just go from day to day." When I asked what that was for her, she explained:

> Chaotic. Things are too chaotic now—the house is chaotic—there is no place I can go just for peace of mind. . . . Foodstamps said that they overpaid me; now I have to pay them back. General Assistance asked what kind of help I'm getting by having my mom here and cut me off. Welfare isn't even interested in you if you don't have a child at home. . . . When times are tough, living day to day is the only thing that pulls me through. When she's [her mother] bad, it's that, well, "Thank god the day is over with," you know, "I made it through the day. Tomorrow's another day, I'll deal with that tomorrow."

Nancy Swenson's situation illuminates the shift from living one day at a time to existing from day to day. Immersion in illness and uncontrollable escalating troubles lead to existing from day to day. What can alter it? An employed spouse, an attentive adult child, a good retirement pension, a comprehensive health insurance policy all provide some protection from having to exist from day to day. Without help, housing, and health care, vulnerability increases dramatically.

More than other men and women, single people and single parents existed from day to day. A middle-aged woman became so debilitated that she had to have help in using the toilet, in taking a bath, etc. Because no insurance program covered her, the tasks fell to her rebellious teen-aged son, who threatened and occasionally hit her. From day to day, she did not know what would happen to her. A mother on welfare lacked the stamina to leave her apartment. She could not monitor her children's activities or protect them from neighborhood gangs. She existed from day to day, overwhelmed by her progressive illness, endless poverty, and fear about what could happen to her children.

When people exist from day to day, the long-term consequences of their health practices seem more distant than they do to other, more fortunate, individuals who have similar conditions. The more locked into the present these people are, the less they will attend to long-term consequences of their actions. John Garston said:

> I'm not thinking all that much about that [his health]. . . . I mean of course I am concerned about it to some degree but, uh, I'm more concerned about today than my long-range health plans. I'm more concerned with getting through today, say, you know dealing with my tensions and worries about other things. I can't be concerned about my long-range health plans when I am concerned with just getting through [the day].

John Garston felt he could handle anything with humor. May Morganson met her problems with equanimity, grateful for having had over forty years of health, unlike the young patients at the dialysis unit. But perhaps for most, existing from day to day means living on the edge—the edge of control, the edge of coping, the edge of desperation.

━━━━━

Mapping a Future

What next? A crisis ends. A treatment works. Existence changes if health and prospects improve. Living one day at a time fades as someone begins to believe that tomorrow will come. Earlier secret hopes and furtive glimpses toward the future now take shape. A future begins to rise on the time horizon. Thus, time perspectives shift to the future. What does that future look like? How do ill people put together a life with a future? What maps of the future do they draw?

Mapping a future means expanding one's time perspective, permitting oneself to plan, and thinking about how to move on the map. When people, particularly single elders, note physical losses, they may include further disability and death in their maps of the future. For most people, however, mapping a future assumes a better future—more control, fewer crises, greater prospects. Mapping a future can give ill people hope, direction, and a sense of control. It may even give them a sense of victory over death. A person may still hope for complete recovery, cure, or reversal in the future. Yet in the meantime, that individual may work toward realizing a future by trying to control illness in the present.

Ill people map different futures at different points in their illness and in their lives. They may map a carefully revised plan for the future, or they may rechart the past, hoping to recapture it. Frequently, people will map routes for making a comeback (Charmaz 1973; 1987; Corbin and Strauss 1988). Yet, maps of the future may remain sketchy; people simply assume that they will realize their futures.

The shape of the map reflects experiences and definitions of illness and how they shift over months and years with mood and bodily feeling. For example, a woman who had breast cancer with lymph node involvement remarked, "I feel my time like a rope—around me—when I feel optimistic, I let it out, the time just unfolds. When I'm feeling pessimistic, the rope is tight." Such shifts can occur rapidly, even within a single conversation. When death is certain, ill people might acknowledge it one moment and then during the next, map a future that extends beyond their most promsing estimations (Charmaz 1980b; Glaser and Strauss 1965; 1968). Five months later, the woman with breast cancer had further metastases. She talked with a friend about her death, expected within months.[4] As they moved on to intellectual topics, she talked of having a future in which she would again explore those ideas. Perhaps at that moment, she recaptured the past and projected herself into a future. Although practitioners may take allusions to a future as illusions and as evidence of denial, claiming a future allows patients some hope and sustains them.

When ill people begin to map a future varies. If aware of the consequences of a crisis or relapse, people with heavy obligations often start while in the midst of it. For example, a single parent said, "I have to figure out a way to go back to school so I can get a desk job later." Similarly, people who have alternatives and are aware of their plights may start sorting through them. An older man commented, "I think I'll just retire—it's only two years early and we've been looking forward to it. I'll sell a piece of property I've had a long time; that'll make up for it."

Others wait to map a future. And wait. They monitor their bodies and their lives. They look for signs to indicate what steps to take next. They map a future or move to the next point on the map only when they feel assured that the worst of their illness is over. These people map a future when they feel distant enough from illness to release their emotions from it. Conversely, if they feel tied to a past illness, they may forego mapping a future. Five years after an episode of Hodgkin's lymphoma, Joanne Dhakzak said:

It suddenly dawned on me, [that] I really don't have any goals— I don't have any goals, per se—nothing concrete. And I was trying to figure out if for the last five years I've been putting myself on hold. "I might not live, so why bother to set goals?" because I might not live long enough to reach the goal.

Now that I'm getting close to the five-year mark in a couple of months, I've *made* it. I'd better set some goals so I have something to work for, otherwise, I'd feel like my life is aimless, and I'd hate it [sighs]. At this point, I feel like I'm bumbling through life as opposed to—"that's my goal and how do I get to my goal?" And it's a terrible feeling and it just dawned on me that maybe it's all connected.

Paths to the future take varied forms. Living one day at a time, for example, dims one's sight of the future, but nonetheless, has consequences for it. Despite her increasing professional success, Sara Shaw did not map a future, but she did take a path, which led to a future. Ten years ago when she was starting her career, she said, "I need to do the maximum that I'm able to comfortably do at any given moment. That includes planning, doing things for the future, but I have no real gut belief—not belief—but I have no real gut security that anything I'm planning exists or will exist."

Four years ago, she had more of a stake in her path to the future, but she did not map set goals:

I know that it's there. And I know that if I wanted to see it, I could. What I ask for now is not to see any big plans of the future, just to let me know what my next step this day is. That's what I want. I want to be living with just a sense of that I am on my right path, that each step that I take is—is working in that direction. And then if I'm off, if something—if I'm going the wrong direction on something, that I'll—just let me get the signals, let them come through. Don't let me deny them; don't let them be shut off from me. . . . So that I can then adjust, you know, and step back on—on track.

Like others, Sara Shaw believed that growing up in an alcoholic family, as well as her illness, kept her time perspective close to the present. Two years ago, she tried to begin to look at a future, while still taking one day at a time. She reflected:

I'm on a real day-to-day right now. . . . It was real hard for me . . . to be able to dream, to have dreams. . . . With the sickness thing, I've really—during that period—really cut off my sense of future dreams because I had to, because I really didn't know if I was going to live. And so that took me a long time. . . . [Lately,] Bob [her fiancé] would talk about something we were going to do and it would just panic me. . . . But I feel like I'm kind of cautiously on a day-to-day, or kind of grounded on a day-to-day and that's very important for me. And that is reality. And then there are things that we can kind of tentatively make plans for. And it's also neat that the idea of making plans totally expecting to accomplish them is different for me because I realize that with my family, plans would be made but you never knew if they were going to happen.

Many people, of course, just live and move into the future as it emerges. They never give it much thought. Joanne Dhakzak described the view she had held of the future throughout her early adulthood: "I never thought of it; I was just plodding along." She had followed her husband around the country and supported his career moves as a naval officer, graduate student, professional, and Ph.D. candidate. Joanne had fit her education and jobs into the cracks of his career choices. She tied the meaning of her illness to finding more purpose in her life:

I feel aimless; so I feel like I have to—for a long time, I felt okay; everything was fine. I was just bumbling around, but it was perfectly fine. But now that's bumbling and I want to have some direction. I don't want to be sixty-five and look back and go, "Well, gee, I've had thirty years that I didn't necessarily have to have and I could have died. I could have been dead by twenty-nine, thirty. I don't want to look back in regret—not regret, but feel like I've wasted my life. It's like I got a second chance and I want to do something with it.

Recapturing the Past

Recapturing the past means that someone hopes to resume past pursuits—and regain a past self. Recapturing the past means far more than restoring lost function or lessened productivity. It means reaffirming the significance of self, both symbolic and actual (Davis 1979; Unruh 1983). Recapturing the past also means being able to interact with others in ways one had in the past. And others may wait and hope for a return of the ill person's past self, which strengthens his or her desire and resolve to recapture the past. For years after her diagnosis of lupus erythematosus, Kathleen Lewis's family hoped to recapture their collective past. She writes:

> My family and I kept taking the "old me" off the shelf, hoping one day she might return and we could go back to our past lives. We'd sigh and put her back on the shelf, but she lingered in our memories and hopes, thwarting any attempts of accepting and living in the present as it was. It was always, "Tomorrow we'll . . ." or "Remember yesterday, when . . . ?" (1985:45)

A desire to recapture the past reflects yearning for a lost self. That yearning results from grieving for accumulated losses from illness. Here, the person defines losses and acknowledges illness. Though she writes that she learned to live moment by moment after her stroke, poet May Sarton simultaneously longed for her past self: "Now I am frightfully lonely because I am *not* my self. I can't see a friend for over a half hour without feeling as though my mind were draining away like air rushing from a balloon" (1988:18).

The sorrow for a past self increases when people believe that they might not reclaim it. Even after trying to wait out illness or treatment, regaining the past self and recapturing the past may remain elusive. Sarton suggests this elusiveness when she writes that "to manage such a passive *waiting* life for so many months I have had to bury my real self—and now realize that bringing that real self back is going to be even more difficult than it was to bury it" (1988:78).

Despite her incapacity, May Sarton's work had taken on a life of its own. Her friends cheered and sustained her. Both work and friends spurred her to regain her health and with it to recapture the past. Further, she had two friends with whom to compare herself; one struggled with depression and the other with frailty. She remarks, "The contrast between these two friends, so much alike in the struggle, and my snail-like existence is ridiculous. I want to be well" (1988:79).

Yearning fades if a renewed self emerges after—or despite—illness. But sometimes no renewal comes, and yearning does not fade. If so, people feel endless sorrow and depression. Then, their nostalgia for a past self intensifies and inundates their images of self founded within diverse involvements. As yearning and nostalgia steadily color one image of self after another, they become etched upon the self-concept.

8

Timemarkers and Turning Points

I was unemployed for four months [this past winter]. . . . It's the only time in my life I ever did not work, other than for health reasons after I got sick. I didn't work for three months [then]. So that was, you know . . . [devastating].

Memorial Day, was my anniversary [the second year after his heart attack], which is not too far back—long ago [three weeks before this interview].

I asked, "What did the anniversary mean to you?" He said:

Oh, time for reflection again. In fact, I went on a bicycle ride. I went half the route that I did go on when I had my heart attack. I wasn't strong enough to go the full twenty-five to fifty miles, so I just did half. I went around to where I had the heart attack, just to see that I could do it. What was I feeling? I don't know—time for reflection—because a lot went on in my life those last two years, you know, economically, health-wise, strain on the family, ah, so—yeah—a lot. How lucky I was [to survive]. . . .

Memorial Day will always mean a time of reflection to me. It always had since Viet Nam. Now with the heart attack, more so. I shall never forget Memorial Day.

Timemarkers and turning points. Mike Reilly marked time by juxtaposing other major events against his heart attack. For him, his heart attack changed everything: work, family, leisure—and health. Three years ago at age forty-two, Mike had achieved an enviable record as a cycling enthusiast. Although never more fit,
196

he collapsed while taking a routine bicycle ride. In an earlier interview, he described his heart attack, the major turning point in his life:

> They were treating me for neck and shoulder injuries and head injuries. Fortunately, I had a helmet. And I was in St. Eugene's [hospital] and they were treating me for that and in the middle of the CAT scan, I had another heart attack and they had to pull me out and ah, put the paddles to me to get my heart going. And then the doctor told me I had a heart attack, and I was just furious about that . . . just—"I'm too young." . . . I was in pretty good shape; in fact, I was almost going to enter a racing circuit for my age group. . . . A bicycle accident I could handle, you know [it's] physical—I've broken my collarbone before, scraped up my legs before—no big deal. But a heart attack seems so final.

Two years afterwards, Mike Reilly remembered his heart attack and the events preceding it with great clarity. But, he remembered fewer details about his hospital stay. When trying to recall those days, he said, "Everything is all blurred to me right now."

What makes some events timemarkers and turning points, but not others? Which events do ill people highlight as part of their chronologies of illness? Which events foreshadow an altered self? Under which conditions do ill people believe that images of self revealed in disturbing events are real? How do they handle their feelings about what happened to them during these experiences?

A timemarker places an event in a chronology. Ill people mark time and note events, which serve as bench marks of a certain direction (Roth 1963). Turning points, however, go beyond bench marks. Not only does a shift in direction result, but also a shift in self follows. Both timemarkers and turning points contribute to constructing a meaningful chronology, and with it, a life history. As ill people search the past to understand the present, they learn about their futures as well as create a chronicle of their illnesses. They bracket certain experiences into distinct events that have form and meaning. These events vary in significance and intensity—from telling moments to all-encompassing episodes, the repercussions of which shape self and reverberate throughout life.

Studying timemarkers and turning points means looking at the past—closely. Beyond serving as points of reference and bench marks of change, feelings about an unsettling or unresolved past event cast shadows on a present self. In the last chapter, I described how ill people related to the present. In this chapter, I shift to the past and look at how markers and feelings shape the past and influence the present.

Illness as a Timemarker

Many people use illness to mark time and to divide periods of their lives (Roth 1963). They celebrate certain markers as anniversaries to note a positive change. Markers can also be cast as comparative anchor points for measuring illness, health and self.

Creating a Chronology

Ill people note how the time within periods of their lives directly relates to self. Their illness chronologies render their experiences more comprehensible. They draw upon their chronologies to help them explain what happened, why they got worse, or better, and what illness meant to them. They also draw upon medical explanations and psychological interpretations like "stress index" that hold cultural currency.

Chronically ill men and women divide their lives into periods of illness and nonillness, crisis and quiescence, flare-ups and remissions, rigid regimens and convalescence. Illness underscores and marks events, and sets boundaries between events. For example, Mark Reinertsen developed a chronology founded on his trials with dialysis and transplant surgery. After he received his second transplant, he felt so much better for several months that he defined being on dialysis as "sick time" and his months with the transplant as "healthy time."

An illness chronology seems like an obvious way to relate to time when sickness has usurped chunks of time, and its effects on self have been glaring. In this case, the chronology of illness seemingly takes on a life of its own. During continued crises or immersion in illness, the chronology overtakes one. Illness shoots by like a train that has left the passenger behind, running after the caboose. Here, the markers of a chronology pile upon one another in such swift succession that they blur together. Moreover, the markers may pose such an assault on one's sense of self that they lie beyond one's ability to take them fully into account. But if people can symbolically or actually keep their illness contained, then they can draw sharp boundaries between their episodes of illness and self.

Establishing a chronology primarily occurs in retrospect. A physician's questions about earlier signs and symptoms, heretofore discounted, can prompt the patient to construct a chronology. Remembering a long discounted and forgotten transitory symptom recasts it as part of one's history. For example, a middle-aged woman had ascertained that her first episode of multiple sclerosis occurred ten years before her diagnosis. She recalled:

> I went blind in one eye. It was right after I'd had Robbie. And that was probably the first time I ever noticed I really had it. . . . I went to run, and all of a sudden it just—you know—there wasn't the energy and everything that I had before wasn't there. And that was in the summer and I think, that was like July, maybe, and come, maybe, September is when I—just all of a sudden this curtain started coming down over my eye. . . . It just came and went and I brushed it off and that was it.

Occasionally, an ill person discerns a pattern when no one else has done so. Decades later, Harriet Binetti felt certain that her first episode of MS occurred when she was in ninth grade. When I asked her what her symptoms were, she said, "Double vision. And I remember my mom just took me to the eye doctor and I wore a patch and they tried to correct it with glasses. And then one day, it just disappeared. And then I didn't have a problem, which was double vision, until I guess early '63."

Another woman who noted her increasingly dry eyes and intensified growing fatigue wondered if she also had Sjögren's syndrome in addition to rheumatoid arthritis. Searching the past helps to explain the present and to predict the future (cf. Katovich 1987). In this way, the chronology develops form and meaning.

These stories underscore a key point: certain events assume more importance in retrospect than when actually experienced. The frame of the emerging chronology gives these past events meaning, whether decreed significant or trivial. An earlier distressing event can seem benign or even positive when juxtaposed against recent ones. Even before her hospitalization, seventy-nine-year-old Carobeth Laird's chronic hip pain, arthritis, inexplicable incoordination, and acute illnesses had confined her. In reevaluating this earlier confinement, she noted:

> I had not felt very secure or very happy in my room in Georgia's mobile home in Chemehuevi Valley. Now I found myself remembering it wistfully. There had been at least a few of my books, some of which had been my companions for years. . . . Now lying in my bed in Indian Hospital, I remembered all these things with nostalgia. Then, in spite of my fears at being left alone while Georgia was away, I enjoyed a comparative freedom and could look forward to a brighter future. Now it seemed unlikely I would ever have a room that I could call my own. (1979:35–37)

When illness serves as a timemarker, people use it as a major source of the stops, hurdles, highs, and lows that give their lives shape and structure. Illness chronologies chart events, specify durations, and locate places and people. They also provide windows for observing the developing self. Through their chronologies, ill people frame experience and thus outline and define feelings as well as physical symptoms. Subsequently, they fill in the spaces of experience between timemarkers (Sharron 1982).

The marker events of a chronology flow from the stance someone takes toward illness. For those who view illness as something to struggle against, the type and duration of the waged battle provide the bench marks of the chronology. Here, the individual constructs a linear chronology to demonstrate progress.[1] Like others, one man relished telling me, "The doctor said, 'You'll never walk again'; [two months later] his jaw dropped a yard when he saw me walking down the hall." Despite grave hardships, handling illness oneself for a period of time without burdening others serves as a timemarker to those who wish to remain stoical. An older woman said, "I got through that bad time and since then, I know I haven't been the same, but I got through it without troubling my relatives or friends."

Illness chronologies are more than markers of time, they also *identify* the individual and establish his or her identity. Early in her chronology, Nancy Mairs developed identity rules about being a person with multiple sclerosis: "Like fat people who are expected to be jolly, cripples must bear their lot meekly and cheerfully. A grumpy cripple isn't playing by the rules. And much of the pressure is self-generated. Early on, I vowed that if I had to have MS, by God I was going to do it well. This is a class act, ladies and gentlemen. No tears, no recriminations, no faintheartedness" (1986: 15).

As I have argued throughout the book, the markers of illness mark self as well as time. And those markers may be seen as positive. As one woman exclaimed, "What I've learned through having this illness is incredible; I like me; I respect me. I have more self-respect than I have ever had." Subsequently, an illness chronology may stand as the history of a transformed self.

If illness becomes special—even precious—to ill people, they see it as a path to self-knowledge. Bench marks in an illness chronology reveal discoveries of self as well as definitions of relative health and illness. "That time [of illness]" takes on intensified meaning and significance. If so, then identifying self with those experiences follows. Other people echoed Sara Shaw's statement: "I wouldn't trade that time [of illness] for anything. Dealing with it made me the person I am today."

Establishing Markers

What are the bench marks of time? Why do some events stand out forever and others blur into the past?

Markers of diagnoses, surgeries, or treatments can serve as anniversary dates, which medical follow-ups and treatments reaffirm. Repeated six-month checkups allow the original marker event to take on weight as both a turning point and reference point. Further, such anniversary dates become part of the daily discourse among patients and families.

When did you have your heart attack?
How long do you have to go until your five-year mark (survival rate)?
It's been three years since diagnosis.
I haven't felt up to par since my surgery five years ago.

Meanings of the anniversary date are often tied to survival.[2] One doctor gave Marty Gordon a prognosis of death within weeks. A year later, she said, "Now that I've had my year anniversary . . . I thought, 'Well, I beat it. There's a year gone by.' And that I feel a lot better than I did and that 'No big deal' and we'll take the next year as it comes."

Certainly the diagnosis and subsequent serious episodes are defined as markers because later events flow from them. What else influences an individual to define an event as a marker?

A family history of an illness can provide ready-made markers for creating comparative chronologies. Mark Reinertsen's mother and uncle had died of the same kidney disease. Several men who had had heart attacks compared themselves to brothers or fathers with heart disease. Two years ago, the doctors of a forty-three-year-old woman thought she had a massive infection due to perforation of the colon. She recounted what the surgeon said: " 'Well, it's definitely not cancer because of your age and everything.' " When I asked her what she knew before she had surgery, she said, "It gets foggy as time goes on, but myself, I knew I had cancer . . . I just kind of had an intuition. Cancer is in my family. My mother's had a mastectomy and my grandfather, her father, died of cancer and I have a cousin who died, oh, three years ago of colon cancer." In addition, this woman's cousin had been about the same age when her colon cancer was diagnosed.

Her family history superseded the initial diagnosis of acute infection and provided grounds for starting her chronology before she received the official news.

The chronology of a relative's unrelated illness may locate and pinpoint events in one's own chronology. For example, Bessie Thompkins located marker events by remembering what was happening to her husband at the same time. "I had the chest pain before Harry went into the hospital—that was three years ago." "Harry was already in St. Eugene's Hospital—before he went to the nursing home—then I had to go into the hospital." Similarly, Lin Bell's brother's sudden fatal heart attack provided the reference point for the beginning of her chronology. She recalled her first episode of angina: "I think it was—let's see, my brother died in '83, so it was April of '83."

Should a hospital stay or a surgical procedure directly precede or follow diagnosis, the marker looms large. A sense of paradox or drama surrounding the initial events strengthens memories of them. Bessie Thompkins said, "Harry and I were both at St. Eugene's at the same time for almost a week. Can you imagine that?" An unexpected crisis with rapid medical intervention provides drama long remembered, and the drama heightens when the medical procedures are risky or if the patient's prognosis remains guarded. For example, one forty-seven-year-old man recounted:

And my wife called the paramedics and. . . . And it took them a week to figure out what was wrong because it's a very rare condition . . . I found out later that it's usually misdiagnosed. The surgeon that did the operation has done, he said something like fifteen hundred bypass operations and this is the third one I think he said that mine was.

It was a high risk procedure, but I didn't really have much choice. . . . They told my wife that—I found out later that they didn't expect me to survive—that they thought they may as well try anyway.

The social consequences of a marker event sharpen the meaning of the event and identify it as a turning point. Several women attributed their broken marriages or relationships to the strain of marker events from illness. The meaning of the marker event thus merges with its social consequences.

The spiraling effects of an illness, in turn, can spawn social marker events such as taking a less demanding job or retiring. These events may mark a changed life, perhaps for an entire family. Mike Reilly's wife had to get her first full-time job in eighteen years, an unwelcome marker for both of them. Lin Bell gave up a job she loved:

> It was a terrific job and I was the only one trained to do it. I was working ten and twelve hours a day, six days a week. That started in '84. And we got this supervisor in—he was not my supervisor—but he kept telling us how things were done in San Tomas, you know, and that we were dumb and didn't know. And I kept telling him, "I don't care how they do it down in San Tomas, get out of my face and let me do my job." And he just kept, just kept it up, just kept it up, 'cause he had other people he wanted in that office. Well he finally got it. I thought, "I don't want to fight." . . . I just want a job that I go to and I leave at work," and so I took a voluntary demotion.

Textbook descriptions of a disease process provide a set of expected timemarkers that signal progression and place ceilings on time. The crucial timemarker estimates death. Given the extent to which she had been affected, Bonnie Presley believed that lupus had foreshortened her life. A middle-aged man who had lived with diabetes for over twenty years said:

> I guess I'm rather pleasantly surprised that I've been a diabetic for so long, with so few bad side effects and I guess the other side of that is I'm kind of apprehensive that ah, before too long, it's going to catch up with me. . . . What I've read about diabetes, it says complications set in after twenty years or twenty-two years or twenty-four years. But I guess I hope that through having to some extent done what I wanted to do, uhm, I kept myself as healthy as I could.

An indeterminate onset obscures the chronology. Certainly having a time limit on life encourages searching the past for the onset of the disease. Without clear timemarkers, people cannot compare their case to a typical one. Nancy Swenson knew that current estimates gave her from two to twenty years to live after the initial onset of symptoms. But when was that? During one interview, when she described herself as sick and depressed, she said, "I figure that I probably had this when I was in Oregon [eight years before]—and possibly before that—if you only live with it as long as twenty years [maximum], I may not have many years left. Whatever time I have left, I'd like it to be peaceful and serene. It's not—I can't get any peace of mind."

As Nancy Swenson's statement implies, the quality of experienced time heightens the significance of timemarkers. And knowing that one has limited time heightens the significance of the quality of time. Several months later, Nancy felt less depressed. At that time, she looked back into the past for timemarkers without the anguish about the present and future. She remarked, "Sometimes I flash back: how long ago was it when I had these first symptoms? [I'm] trying to figure out how much longer, you know, if I live to the max of what that says I'm going to have. . . . Sometimes I think about, God, *that* was a sign, and *that* was a sign of the carcinoid, you know, but nobody picked up on it."

Vague symptoms without a legitimizing diagnosis can give rise to a chronology based more upon nasty encounters with physicians than on symptoms or episodes. An older woman challenged several doctors' assertions about her and ultimately was refused treatment by the only specialist in town. Her chronology consisted of the sequence of her hostile encounters with physicians.

What, when, and how people mark events connected with illness depend upon their awareness of it, other pressing concerns, and their degree of attachment to it. An older man gave a much more detailed chronology of his wife's illness than of his own, which he discounted as rather uninteresting. But once illness has consumed someone's interest and governs his or her days, a response like this is common: "Why I can tell you every little detail. I mean I have stories that could bore you to death."

Markers as Measures

When people mark time by illness, what do the markers mean? What lies between the marked events? By comparing views of self in illness with other views of self, one can measure the present self. Measures can be taken of how "sick" or "well" the person is. Similarly, marking time prospectively takes a different cast than finding retrospective markers. Prospective markers can focus effort, such as when someone prepares to go back to work or aims to walk a specific distance by a projected date. But what occurs between retrospective markers often seems elusive, because losing one's health can occur slowly. In these circumstances, markers emerge and measure physical changes only when the person becomes aware of lost function.

When she was very ill, Bonnie Presley remarked, "Well, I think about the past when, like you know, if my hand won't turn on the knob in the shower . . . or my arm is so tired I can't brush my teeth, sure I think about 'Gosh, remember when I used to be like this and that and do this and that.' "

Retrospective markers can also flag the road back to health. Thus, a prior ill self serves as the contrast for measuring present self and marks the distance that has been covered. Mike Reilly said:

> 1987 I would say was the worst year of my life, economically, financially, stress-wise and all that. So I'll mark time by that. You know, five years ago I did this. What were you doing? God, it's been five years since my heart attack. And also, it's when things are bad, you know, what's the worst you ever felt? I can move back to that and, "Look what I've accomplished since that." So I use that, try and use it from a positive point of view.

A marker event is distinct and even extraordinary. Yet markers can change. A once distinct event blurs when repeated without change. An initial hospitalization, for example, stands as a marker since people define it as a turning point, a vivid symbol of change. However, if frequent subsequent hospitalizations do not produce much change, they grow routine—unless, of course, one hospitalization is a long-awaited evaluation at a leading medical center (Gross 1987).

Markers are not merely reconstructions after the events. Ill people actively construct markers and chronologies in the midst of crisis and uncertainty as well (Roth 1963). They mark events while immersed in illness to note improvement and to provide a way of measuring the next hurdle. Joanne Dhakzak said, "I built a situation to get through it and then used it as an anchor to get through the next one." Her situations ranged from markers during the day to major goals. For example, if she got her dogs walked in the morning, then, she reasoned, she could get herself to treatment that day. Similarly, with a longer timeframe: "If I could get through radiation, then I could handle chemotherapy." She used the marker to measure what and how much to do next.

Markers hold less encompassing meaning if ill people believe that the worst is over. Then, they treat events as markers but refer to them as they will. They pull up parts of their pasts as though files on a computer, catalog them, review their contents, and then, perhaps, clear them from memory.[3] Joanne Dhakzak commented, "Before, everything revolved around illness. Now I want to treat it as something I learned from, a growth experience, something that I developed from—treat it as a measuring—a marker."

Identifying Moments

Some timemarkers seem objective and external. In contrast, identifying moments and significant events are existential. They touch the self directly. Identifying moments are telling moments filled with new self-images. And they are telling because they spark sudden realizations, reveal hidden images of self, or divulge what others think.

Some identifying moments are positive. For example, an older woman with cancer surprised and delighted an elderly man with heart disease by saying, "The way you have handled your illness has been such an inspiration to me; you are my role model."

Yet many identifying moments astonish or demean the ill person. Like the small shocks of awareness of aging (Karp 1988), unsettling reminders of a changing self and a new identity can emerge when one loses his or her health. An elderly woman almost fell after using the toilet. She said, "I realized then my days of living independently are numbered." A man with heart disease suddenly saw how much his heart attack had aged him. He commented: "When I went to this exercise class with Janie—Janie Neilson—um, they had mirrors around the gymnasium and ah, we were doing exercises, walking around the perimeter of the gymnasium, and I looked at myself in the mirror and I said, 'You know, I can't really believe I'm that old, to have all these problems,' and I really felt depressed."

Practitioners often create identifying moments, sometimes intentionally. Lin Bell recalled her first heart attack. She said, "And then, I woke up in CCU [cardiac care unit] and there's Janie [the cardiac rehabilitation nurse] bending over me, saying, 'Congratulations for quitting smoking.' " Later, when she was enrolled in the cardiac rehabilitation program, Lin dismissed the fears that other patients had. Again, Janie, her program leader, provided several identifying moments:

> When I was exercising, see, I wasn't real worried about myself because I'd only had angioplasty. Most of these people there had had bypasses or heart attacks and they had pacemakers and all that. Not me, I only had angioplasty. And Janie kept telling me, "Lin, you'd better watch out," you know. Then she knew I was smoking again. She said, "Your second heart attack, you have a 50 percent chance of it being fatal." I said, "No sweat, Janie; I haven't had my first one yet." And she said, "You had angioplasty; that is considered like a heart attack." I thought, "Well, criminy."

Commonly, invisible illnesses evoke identifying moments because others discount people's claims to illness or accuse them of exaggerating. Noticeable disabilities elicit a different order of identifying moments. Even strangers make intrusive comments or ask rude questions. Harriet Binetti remarked in disgust about "the pity disabled people get in wheelchairs and you know, they're always [saying] "hi" [mimicks the condescending tone]. You get that smile. . . . You're walking down the street [in her electric wheelchair], some guy stopped his car and got out and put his hand on my shoulder and wanted to pray for me. Yeah, it's a weird world. And they look at *me* as though I'm weird."

If ill people hold strong positive views of themselves and their conditions, they are likely to reject the negative messages within the identifying moment. Marty Gordon, who had idiopathic pulmonary fibrosis, said, "People who know me well, can hear me breathe; it's like a pant. You could tell. Every once in a while someone will say that I'm breathing that way to get attention. That's their denial. They aren't able to deal with it. I just let it go; it doesn't bother me. I just say to myself, "That's okay—they can't deal with it; that's just their way of reacting."

In contrast, the labels stick when significant or powerful others undermine or negate a person's taken-for-granted assumptions about self. These identifying moments elicit consternation and grief. The moment escalates into an identifying crisis and, likely, becomes a lasting significant event and turning point (Charmaz 1980a). Like a building in a severe earthquake, the self is shaken and wrenched from its assumed foundation. The self now requires reconstruction, not simply reappraisal. Here, the boundaries between an identifying moment, identifying crisis, significant event, and turning point merge.

Ernest Hirsch saw himself as a psychotherapist who happened to have multiple sclerosis. He writes:

When I noticed that no patients were being assigned to me, I made an appointment with the new director. I went to his office completely without suspicion, altogether unaware of the bomb that was about to be exploded in my face. . . . The chief of this service, looking highly uncomfortable, said that I would not be assigned any more patients. He explained that, because of my illness, patients might feel sorry for me, so that I could not have optimal effectiveness as their therapist. . . . This pronouncement came altogether unexpectedly. I hadn't even vaguely thought that anything of this sort was in the air and, truth to tell, didn't think that anyone had given any special thought or notice to my illness. No one hardly talked about it at all. But I found out that I was simply to finish the psychotherapy cases that I was carrying and that I was then to end my psychotherapeutic activities for good and all. What had been at the center of my professional life was no longer to be even at the periphery. I could not imagine what my professional life, or even just my life, would be like without doing this type of work. (1977:71–72)

Significant Events as Turning Points

Relived moments. Retold stories often evoke recurring feelings. Significant events echo in memory. Whether validating or wholly disrupting, a significant event reveals images of present or possible self and evokes feelings. Thus, these events mark time and become turning points.

A significant event stands out in memory because it has boundaries, intensity, and emotional force. Furthermore, a significant event captures, demarks, and intensifies feelings. Frequently, those feelings are unhappy ones such as bewilderment, humiliation, shame, betrayal, or loss. The event flames and frames these feelings. The emotional reverberations of a single event echo through the present and future and therefore, however subtly, shade thoughts and feelings about self and alter meanings of time (cf. Denzin 1984).

Significant events transcend the actors within them and the stage on which they occur. These events are emergent realities, events *sui generis;* they cannot be reduced to component parts (Durkheim 1951). Thus, a significant event reflects more than a relationship or another's actions. When, where, and how the event occurs and who participates in it contribute to the force of the event and affect subsequent interpretations of it. Sorting out what the event means and the "correct" feelings to hold about it shapes self-images and self-worth.

A significant event freezes and enlarges a moment in time. Because of inherent or potential meanings of self within the event, people grant obdurate qualities to it. They reify it. To them, the event supersedes past meanings and foretells future selves.

Like Ernest Hirsch, my respondents had to make sense of shocking, disturbing, and ambiguous events. They had to handle their recurring feelings about the self that were reflected in the event. How did they do it? By reliving and retelling these events. And in doing so, they gained new perspectives on ambiguous or distressing events and on themselves. Original meanings of positive significant events, however, were retained, as the following stories indicate.

Finding Positive Events

Some events connected with illness are positive or come to be defined as such. People savor positive significant events while experienced and long relive and retell them. These events engender pride and may alleviate earlier shock, self-blame, or shame. For example, a young woman had blamed herself for her pain and other people had agreed that she should. Learning of another interpretation without self-blame was a revelation to her:

> I took a class in existentialism. . . . [The professor] said, "Pain is the experience of having a body." Instead of it being *my* fault, it was simply the experience of having a body and it didn't have to be self-deprecating. That made a lot of sense to me. I could just feel the pain and say, "Yeah, feel that pain, so I am alive and I have a body," and I could go on. And from that moment forward—that was a real "Aha!" period for me—the disease just cleared up—that particular class and that particular piece of information as well as others changed my life a great deal.

This woman then was able to believe that she could have a life beyond pain. My respondents spoke of other positive significant events such as comforting another anxious patient, finishing a crucial task despite being ill, or realizing that one no longer had to face crises or deal with negative feelings seen in another person.

These events take on significance because ill people view them as turning points that mirror growth and resiliency of self.

In addition, these events affirm that one has taken control over illness, rather than the converse. The positive event itself becomes a turning point for subsequent positive events. Goldie Johnson's health had plummeted. Within six years, she could only move around her living room in her electric wheelchair. For her first seventy-two years, she had been a leader in her lodge and church. As her disability increased, she grew more angry and bitter. She felt cheated because she was so physically limited. She viewed not only her dancing days as over, but also her social life. Goldie wondered if life was worth living at all. Her dark thoughts faded after a near-death experience recast the present and future. When I asked her what she felt upon being revived, she said:

> I felt good because I heard the Lord's voice. In the room where they took me, I could see these windows like these [the picture window facing her] and the nurse said to me, "Turn over on your shoulder," so I was turning and saw the light coming in. I heard a voice [saying], "You can stay. I've got work for you to do." Oh, it was the most beautiful voice you'd ever hear. I started to fight and I woke up. . . . I'm glad to be back. I'm trying to figure out what He wants me to do. . . .
> I still sit here and wonder about that voice.

Goldie Johnson's daughter testified to the change in her mother's outlook after this experience. She said, "It's like night and day. She was so down before; she'd given up. Now she's like she used to be." Life had a purpose again for Goldie Johnson.

Turning points occur when ill people learn that they can give to others who suffer. Gilda Radner had a breakthrough event when she first talked in her cancer support group. She reclaimed her lost self and, simultaneously, learned that she could help other members:

> And then one day I opened up and said, "My name is Gilda Radner and I am a performer by trade. When I got cancer it appeared on the cover of the *National Enquirer*. They said, 'Gilda Radner in Life-Death Struggle,' and since then everybody has thought I was dead. Well, I'm not dead—cancer doesn't have to mean you die."

Everyone in the room was looking at me a little more closely. It was as though at that moment I became Gilda Radner. I got very funny as I told stories about going to a restaurant and seeing someone back up against the wall because he was so frightened to see me. "I don't know if he was upset because I was alive or because he didn't send me a card."

At the end of the meeting a lot of the women came up to me asking questions like "What kind of chemo are you on?" "What happened when your hair fell out?" And I saw that they were looking to me for answers or leadership. I tried to help and say what I felt. (1989: 144–145)

Past events may be recast and reconstructed in light of their positive consequences. The initial events surrounding an illness, for example, had once been thought of as multiple disasters. Later, they may become redefined as turning points toward a more aware self and positive markers of deeper meanings and changed involvements.

Marker events may not always stem from the person's illness, although they can be reminders of mortality. Vera Mueller's sister died suddenly of undiagnosed heart disease at thirty-five. Vera's shock and grief became the pivotal marker in her life:

Cynthia's death—I cannot—I cannot begin to explain what happened to me in the moment . . . the woman that I had never talked to in my life . . . identified herself, and she said, "Vera dearie, I hate to be the one to tell you this, but your sister died." And I screamed. I screamed. I was so angry. I mean it was just—there was never anything but pure, pure, fundamental, I don't know what the word—primal anger pouring out of me over the telephone. I just—I let loose with—Oh! Did I ever let loose. And I never let go of it . . . and then after her death, I went through the whole process of looking at my life and getting with those feelings. . . . One of the things Cynthia's death did for me was allow me the opportunity to stand back and say, "Wait a minute, Vera, are you somebody? Who do *you* think you are? What do you believe?" And then to say, "Well, by God, if you believe it, you'd better get on living it because you might be the one to go next.

By facing her sister's death, Vera Mueller faced herself. By taking this stance, she transformed what had seemed a tragic, meaningless death into the turning point that let her take a different, positive path. She avowed:

> I mean Cynthia's death is *the* turning point at this point. Everything before that had been luck, happenstance, and swimming around in a quagmire of confusion and lack of understanding. And I don't blame myself for that. There is no blame to be placed anywhere. It just was the way it was. And since that time, I have been doing everything from the time I get up in the morning until I go to bed at night, to put my life together.

Reliving Negative Events

Negative events are relived and, often, retold time and time again. Crushing moments. Humiliating encounters. Betrayal. As Ernest Hirsch's (1977) story implies, ill people can feel crushed, humiliated, and betrayed during a single event. Through the event, someone's assumptions about life, health, relationships, and self can be knocked asunder. Harry Bauer said, "I think my biggest blow was when I was told to either retire or get my box [casket]. And that wasn't all that easy to live with." Though ten years had passed since his retirement, he still felt the loss of his work. He said, "I cope with it."

Events filled with shame are less likely to be retold, but perhaps, more likely to be relived—over and over and over. These events call into question both bodily functioning and a competent self. Hence, evident impotence, incontinence, or memory lapse spawn long remembered shame. Ann Rorty's episodic bowel incontinence caused several nightmarish incidents:

> I had Levi's on and I had a little bit of an accident before I got off the bus. So as soon as I got into Green's [drugstore], I had to run back to the bathroom. I had to sit in there and clean myself up. Used a whole bunch of toilet paper and of course if someone wanted in . . . [raises hands to indicate, "What could I do?"]. And then I was going to do some shopping but all I did was go

over and get my drugs and split as fast as I could. And I was shaking. I was torn apart.

Shame lasts. As Izard (1977) notes, shame involves a heightened consciousness of self and implies failure. It strips away self-respect. The person feels reduced and ridiculed (cf. Lewis 1971). When shame touches a shaky self, it can encompass the self and paralyze feeling.[4] Under these conditions, shame reflects a fundamental uncertainty about both self-definition and self-worth. And that uncertainty is precisely what having serious chronic illness and disability can evoke (Brody 1987). Consequently, significant events founded in shame echo for months and years after.

In contrast, shocking events that threaten loss of control or life are long remembered, but they lose intensity over time—particularly if one lives. At fifty-eight, Marty Gordon had been hospitalized for extensive tests. Eight months later, she told this story:

He [the doctor] came in to tell me, "Uh, it didn't look good and that this was a—could be a very rapidly"—and it appeared that mine was really going rapidly and it might be about six weeks. Whoa! That blew my mind. It really did. And I think again, in hindsight, he did not do it right—but he was the statistician, it wasn't Dr. Schultz [her rheumatologist]. Right after that—I'm a Catholic—right after that, a poor little volunteer lady came in and [said], "Mrs. Gordon?" And the doctor had said, "Mrs. Gordon" "Yeah, OK." And then he told me. She said, "I'm from St. Mary's Church." I said, "Jesus, Mary, and Joseph, they've got the funeral already." And it really just—then I began to see humor in it, but I was scared. And I think that night was my biggest night. . . .
   I had my cry. I read a chapter [of *Love, Medicine, and Miracles*]. And I flipped on Joan Rivers . . . and was hysterical [with laughter]. All by myself. And I think that this was the point when—[I decided], "If this is going to happen OK, but I'm not going to let it happen." . . . And I think probably that was the turning point when I said I wouldn't accept it. You know, I will not accept that uhm, death sentence, or whatever you want to call it. And ah, I think since then I've been going uphill instead of downhill.

Progressive loss of control can turn an otherwise annoying but inconsequential incident into a significant event and a turning point in stance and action. Christine Danforth sought a physician who could alleviate her discomfort. However, she could ill-afford the money that her search cost since her low-paying jobs did not provide health insurance. She went to four different physicians, each of whom charged her hefty initial fees and ordered complete and costly X-rays and lab tests. Her story reveals how the meaning of a significant event builds on past events:

> I would go in for the second visit and they would [each] say, "Yes, you have lupus, what do you want me to do?" And I would say, "I want you to do something. I'm not comfortable, something's wrong." They would never tell me what to do. . . . I called and talked to her [the fifth doctor] on the phone and I said [that] I've been diagnosed with lupus, and I said, "I want you to tell me on the phone if you can't help me; I don't want to waste my time, my money, and your time." And she said, "Oh, no," you know, "I have lupus patients, I can help you." And I said, "OK fine." I went in for a visit. It was $90. She said, "I need you to have these tests taken." And I said, "I just had all of those done two weeks ago." I said, "Can't you use those?" "No, I need a new set." I said, "But these are only two weeks old." And she said, "No, I need them again." So I went in and I had them all taken again, which was another couple hundred dollars. . . .
>
> I had no insurance. I went back to her for my second time after she got the results back and maybe she had a bad day and I had a bad day, but I walked in and she said, "Yes, you have lupus, what do you want me to do?" And I blew [up]. I just came unglued. I just—I came unglued. And she said, "Well, that's your problem, right there; it's your attitude." And I just said, "Attitude, hell lady; you don't know what attitude is." And she was like, you know, the fifth one down the line and I was just furious. So she said, "Well, I don't know what you want me to do or what you expect me to do?" and I—just nothing, you know, and I walked out and she said, "Well, you make an appointment on your way." And I didn't and I left. And she called me the next day at work and said, "Well, I see you didn't make an appointment." And I said, "It's useless, you know. If you feel my prob-

lem is my attitude, then there's no use even to continue it." So I never went back.

The culminating sense of betrayal, frustration, anger, and loss of control that Christine Danforth felt was echoed in other men's and women's stories. Loss of control alone can cause ill people to relive and retell the event because it can elicit such profound questions. Loss of control increases when someone already feels a lack of control in key relationships. Christine had tried to exert some control over her medical care. This last medical encounter not only echoed her lack of control in all the previous encounters, but also symbolized her lack of control over her care and her health. A sense of loss of control intensifies when ill people believe that a conceivably unrelated event actually turns on their being ill. Tina Reidel retold this story several times:

And the worst thing that ever happened. . . . They [her lover and his son] just took my stuff [to store it] and threw it in the car and went over to my house . . . that I'd rented out to the tenants. . . . When I'd try to put the key in the door to my house . . . none of the keys fit and we couldn't get into the house. So Jim [her lover] said that he was going to sit there until someone came home. And he had a real asthma attack from the old moldy stuff. So I got hysterical . . . and I phone up his [Jim's] daughter-in-law and [told her where the tenant worked] . . . and I said, "Get the key from him," so she went out and he wouldn't give the key to her and ah, he told her his girlfriend's address . . . and I could get the key from her. This was so humiliating; I'd never met this woman before; *she* had a key to my house. And I didn't have a key to my own house and so I—like everything was out of control. And we just took all this stuff and threw it into the basement. . . . *It's like a total loss of control. Because of the arthritis, I couldn't deal with anything* [emphasis mine].

I just think these people really took advantage of me, you know, like his son—Jim's son—and the tenants in my house, and everyone—like I had no power and no control or anything and that was because of the arthritis, because it was so overwhelming, just the arthritis, just to deal with my own body.

218 ■ ILLNESS, THE SELF, AND TIME

For Tina Reidel, loss of control of her health spread to loss of control of her life. To others, loss of identity within the events spreads to an identifying crisis that lasts. Still evincing sorrow, loss, shame, and betrayal after eight years, a young woman revealed that a previous stepfather had taunted her about her incoordination (Charmaz 1973; 1980). His taunts culminated in the identifying crisis that she relived and retold as we talked. My field notes state:

> With just the mention of the stepfather [she] became visibly more upset. Her facial grimacing increased as did her extraneous move-ments. She said, "My brother was married by then and he thought I should have it [a dwindling inheritance from their father] for the car since I had such a hard time at home." By this time she was close to breaking down and her movements were even more uncontrolled. "My stepfather didn't like me—he was always making fun of my coordination." I asked how long the family had lived with her stepfather. She said (while reaching a height of grimacing and extraneous movements), "He tried to strangle me. I haven't seen him since." (Charmaz 1973: 66)

As she retold the event, she relived the same feelings she had experienced eight years before. Her emotions remained tied to definitions of self experienced in the event, but not to her stepfa-ther, whom she had dismissed. Her humiliation and shame resulted in self-doubt and low self-esteem and had remained with her for eight years. The event evoked "feeling reminders" (Hochschild 1979). In her eyes and also, she believed, in the eyes of any reasonable human being, her present self still re-mained a diminished self.

Here, present experience and sense of self reflect the feelings founded in a past self-image. The distance from past to present shrinks as the past flashes into the present (Goffman 1963; Scheler 1961). The person relives the emotions of the past. Con-tinued reexperiencing of the original emotion etches it deeper into the structure of the self (Scheler 1961). Further, a dramatic event that first elicits correct "social" responses, such as shock or anger, over time may be transformed into a psychological event dredged up in memory with haunting "personal" emo-tions such as grief or shame.

In the story above, the woman believed that the meaning of the event was clear. In contrast, other ill people relived and retold an event to self and others to establish their stance on it. They told it to receive another "take" on its meaning. The original event raised identity questions that long remained unresolved. Consequently, by telling and retelling, they develop, solidify, and reify a stance on the event, on themselves in the event, and on their future selves. Sara Shaw explained, "In the telling and retelling each time, I gain perspectives and understand more fully what happened during that time. That helps me decide what to do from here." Ultimately, then, telling and retelling can help to gain closure on the event.

The self-images mirrored in the event demand serious thought. Even though the looking-glass self (Cooley 1902) might reflect a "distorted" image, conceivably a shocking one, it foretells a possible self.

Relived and retold events flood consciousness, shape views, and provide a frame for juxtaposing present events, feelings, and meanings. No friends visited Mark Reinertsen during his first transplant surgery, which saddened him. In subsequent months, he made detailed plans to ensure that friends would be there during his second transplant attempt. His strategies failed. After the second transplant surgery, he disclosed:

> I didn't have any people that I cared about come visit me while I was in the hospital, any of my friends up here. . . . And I thought about that and I said, "Well, OK, it's a long drive and some people don't like to go to hospitals." But I didn't receive letters from them, I didn't receive phone calls from them. . . . Found out afterwards that most of them did know. The men in my Men Against Violence group, none of them. And what happened is the day that I got called, I phoned one of them and told him, "Let the word out that I'd like to hear from people while I'm down there." And he didn't.

Retelling allows people to discover nuances within the event, to draw them out, and to scrutinize them. Because retelling leads to deciding on a view of reality, it shapes actions and emotions.

Ill people may hold seemingly contradictory stances on the event. They may feel angry, yet simultaneously still feel attached to the event. It marks the beginning of their present selves. Afterwards, these people take pride in handling an earlier negative event successfully. They gain positive continuity of self over time (cf. Marris 1974). By examining the past, they resolve problems within it (cf. Marshall 1980; Strauss 1964). Sometimes, they look back in awe at their own courage and strength. Facing the event can result in revelations about themselves and their lives. Mark Reinertsen discovered that handling his harrowing experiences with illness reduced his fear and dread:

> Experiencing illness is never as bad as it seems. *Never* as bad as it seems. Uh, I—I would say, "oh, my God, this is terrible." And then in the meantime, someone would come along, and he'd be ten times worse and, oh see? And not just in that sense, but also in the sense that I can always go around and find someone else who's having to struggle too and even people who are healthy have struggles. And it is important not to get caught up in that melodrama.

Present Emotions and a Past Self

Reliving and retelling significant events can lead to experiencing present emotions through the images, judgments, and appraisals of self implied or proclaimed in the past event. Here, past views of self circumscribe and define present feelings. Present and future become melded with the past. As Cooley (1902) observed, sentiments and feelings form foundations for the self and also result in measures of self-esteem. Retelling the event becomes a means of sorting, defining, and clarifying old sentiments that constitute the self. Hence, an ill person may do considerable "emotion-work" (Hochschild 1979) to understand present feelings in relation to a past self.

A person with an already fragile self-concept likely accepts negative judgments and images of self revealed in a significant event. Then, the event raises feelings that merge with self

(Denzin 1980). The questions that arose in the event pervade present self and feelings. To illustrate: a woman discovered that her physician, whom she adored, believed that she was malingering. Feeling reduced in his eyes prompted a tearful, tense encounter, which became a turning point. For three years after, she discounted her symptoms saying to herself, "I'm just overreacting." When symptoms worsen, but the meanings of the earlier event last, ill people ask questions like: "Did I bring this episode on myself?" "Do I want to be sick?" "I wouldn't have it, would I, if my head was in a better place?"

When an earlier significant event reverberates in these ways, people remain in the past, in past emotions and relationships, though chronological time moves on. They come to define emotions and meanings of the past as "true" and "real." And then, this self-image reflected by the past becomes their "real" self (cf. Turner 1976).

As Denzin (1984) notes, people with dominant negative emotions remain frozen in the present as they resurrect the past. Yet, these ill people may not have always dwelt on negative feelings. The significant event becomes the turning point when their feelings shifted. Initially surreal, shocking events become plausible or even "true." For example, a young woman retold an encounter with a psychiatric resident during her hospital stay:

> If my boyfriend came and left and I was in tears, he immediately shows up like: young doctor enter stage left. It was horrible. . . . He felt I had been coming on to him sexually and, therefore, he wanted to refer me to someone else. . . . I mean I was *not* sexually attracted to him. But I also remember that I didn't argue with him. You know, if it were me today I would just say something obscene to him or something . . . that it was definitely his problem, and he might want to take a look at it. . . . He was a professional who definitely blew it. Even though *I knew* in my heart that I was not coming on to him sexually . . . I was in such a bad place with myself that I thought, "Well, maybe I am, maybe I am, I don't know it." But—I mean I know myself well enough *now* to know that if you don't think you are and you're not attracted to a person, that you are not. You know, it's simply that. But nothing was very simple to me then and I figured well—here he was, a

professional—he should know. He's probably right. So that I think he did me a lot of damage in that case.

At that time, she had viewed her illness as one more failure, culminating in this doctor's pronouncements. Hence, his definition of her feelings became difficult for her to contradict. It took years for her to counter those feelings of failure and to reestablish positive feelings about self. In effect, the subjective duration of the event and the negative feelings lengthen and supersede other concerns.

Such events weigh on an ill person's mind like a prison sentence on a defendant who had expected acquittal. The more isolated, lonely, inactive, and dependent someone is, the more influence these events have, particularly when powerful or intimate others suggest the "proper" self-images and emotions for the ill person to have. One astute physician observed that his elderly patients took his offhand, casual, or flippant remarks as absolute authority and a direct reflection upon them.

When facing ambiguity, power plays an especially important role in feeling and defining emotions (Kemper 1978). Implicit or explicit feeling directives from powerful others provide frameworks for "understanding" and experiencing self and situation, even when these frameworks demean or devalue oneself.

Many ill people do not know what to feel. Frequently, their experiences are ambiguous and they face them without allies. Ill people *experiment* with both their feelings and actions (Tavris 1982). And, their feelings are often mixed. For example, someone may simultaneously feel fear about the prognosis, anger about incomplete information, self-pity for being ill, envy toward those who are not, inadequate for being dependent, and gratitude for receiving care. Which feeling becomes defined as the overriding, defining emotion in an event depends on the person's vulnerability, the intensity of the experience, the relative power of people who control it, and the meanings that the person attributes to others. Later, an ill individual, especially with the help of others, may define one emotion as his or her "true" feeling about the entire event.

Significant events frequently elicit past feelings and doubts. For those respondents who blamed themselves for their illnesses and, moreover, for earlier problems in their lives, the significant event takes on ominous proportions. It "reflects" and magnifies all prior failings. Sara Shaw had ruminated about why her mother hadn't visited her very often when she was immersed in illness. In an interview three years after that period, she said, "I felt like it must be my—it must be something wrong with me, or it must be my fault that my own family didn't even want to deal with me, you know, when I was dying. So I felt like, you know, I felt real guilty, like I must be real bad, or I must have done something real bad for my mother, like, to shun me."

Sara Shaw's emotions remained anchored in the events of the past. As a result, her private self remained in a past where all her doubts concerning self-worth continually reemerged, even though she had developed a confident professional self.

After years of self-blame and guilt, followed by sadness and anger, Sara Shaw felt afraid to trust others. When she discussed her ambivalance about finding someone to love, she discovered that her emotions remained tied to the past. During our conversation, she suddenly realized that she had worked on improving everything but her emotions:

No wonder! Sara, [to herself] no wonder. I *want* to like people but I am *so* scared to. Like right now I feel like I want to cry. . . . I never would have thought that this [trust] was a part of the whole thing of being sick, I never would have thought it—I was so determined—once that I [had] decided I was going to live regardless of anybody else or anything else. Then I thought I'd hit most of the bases and uh, this just threw me for a loop to discover this [that she had not dealt with her feelings about intimacy and trust].

Sara Shaw's remarks suggest the elusive nature of defining and managing feelings resulting from the significant event. She was aware of hurt, anger, loss, and betrayal during the event and clearly aware of the event itself. She also knew how to manage her life afterwards in order to have more control over it. Yet, the crucial area of intimacy had remained hidden and elusive to her for over five years.

Unless people redefine or transform their feelings about a significant event that diminished them, they can remain tied to meanings and sentiments of these past events. Even if their health greatly improves, these people retain a crucial link to a past period of illness, which the event marks and symbolizes. Past, present, and future become inextricably linked in their hidden feelings, although the past may be left behind in other, more visible, parts of their lives.

Transcending Past Emotions

Transcending the negative emotions of past events can occur implicitly if people can develop new lives. New social worlds offer chances for new self-images. New friends or lovers may buttress an emerging sense of worth. Achievement at school or work provides "evidence" for redefining feelings about self, such as a prior conviction that one cannot function.

Usually it takes months or years to transcend low self-esteem symbolized in emotions about a significant event, especially when these emotions have melded with the self-concept. If this happens, later single "successes" do not wield as much power over self-definition as one earlier negative significant event. Rather, it takes many successes, and much evidence of positive value, before one can discard earlier negative feelings and shift views of self. Although transcending the emotions of the past usually occurs imperceptibly, some people redefine "correct" emotions and eventually reject the feeling directives in the significant event.

When people reject feeling directives, they refuse to allow them to merge wholly with their self-concepts. If they have power or disregard the other's power, they may try to impose a view of reality and to influence others' actions.

To do so, they reopen the earlier event and ask others to reappraise it. An ill person may then demand that others relive it as he or she has relived it in haunting memories. Reexamining the original event can raise new questions and challenge earlier moral meanings. With these questions, anchors to the past loosen and new possibilities for the present and future arise. For example, when a person comes to believe that anger, indignation, or amusement might be more appropriate emotional responses to an earlier event than shame or resignation, he or she has also challenged the dictates of earlier moral meanings.

When Sara Shaw began to reject her earlier emotional alignment with the events of five years before, she confronted her family about them. She recounted the tense family scene in these words:

> I got everybody together and sat down and I just got hysterical, like I just started crying a whole lot, and I just said, "Where were you guys?" [when she was seriously ill], you know, "Why weren't you there? What was going on with all of you?" And I told them that I needed to know this, if I was going to . . . be a part of the family, that I needed to know what happened during that time with them and why they weren't there . . . when I got to the point where I didn't know if I was going to be able to take care of myself. The doctor started saying [then], "Do you have any family? Where are they? We have to contact them now." . . . And so I sat down and I wrote a letter to my mom and I said, "In the event that I get to the point where I cannot take care of myself, can I come home?" And she wrote me a letter back and she said, "No, you can't come home, because you don't get along with your father."

Sara Shaw forced her family to deal with her present feelings about the past event, whether or not they dealt with the past event itself. Through reopening the past, she gained more information and insight about it. She discovered that her brother actually had not known how sick she had been. She learned more about her position in the family and simultaneously found a possibility of recasting her role within it. She created a scene in order to teach her family to accept her views of her moral rights and to acknowledge the legitimacy of her emotional response to the past event. Doing so strengthened her claims to reinterpreting the "true"—i.e., unjust—meaning of the past. During the ensuing confrontation, Sara's sister tried to elicit Sara's guilt and self-blame for causing a fuss and for hurting their mother. But Sara refused to accept her sister's definitions of "correct" feelings. Instead, she felt that the balance of suffering had been righted. She recounted that she told her sister, "I've paid my dues, you know, I went through enough pain, and go ahead, give me all the guilt you want."

Momentarily, at least, Sara Shaw controlled interaction, and probably the emotional climate, within her family (Becker 1975). Shame, sorrow, and loss from the past were transformed into anger and indignation. Similarly, what had been an obsessive review became the source of moral action and legitimate redress. These feelings and meanings reflect a self now less vulnerable to others' judgments (Kemper 1978; Tavris 1982). Paradoxically, such an appraisal of the significant event can itself become another significant event, although in Sara's case, a positive one.

Once committed to a revised version of the significant event, the person may insist that other participants' feelings and actions should logically flow from these new definitions (Becker 1960) and events. Vera Mueller assumed her son owed her a modicum of good behavior. Although she had never told him of the seriousness of her condition, she revealed it to him when his violent threats toward other children thoroughly provoked her. She explained:

> I didn't put my life on the line for him to act like a little shithead. His eyes popped out [when she said that]. He said, "What do you mean?" I said, "They told me to have an abortion, I told them to go to hell." [She now recounts her son's question]: "Why did you tell them that?" [She responded to him]: "Because they told me that it would kill me for you to be born. I told them they were wrong. I *fought* for you to be brought into this world before you were even here. How dare you turn around and do something that stupid?"

These two stories reflect different uses of reopening the event that occur along the same continuum. In the first story, Sara Shaw raised questions about the earlier event. Reopening it meant discovering what had happened, checking impressions, and deciding which feelings to hold about family. As a result, one may redefine large slices of time. In the second story, however, the meaning of the significant event remained firm. No clarifying or reexamining needed here. Instead, reopening the event was used to exact specific actions from another individual.

The effects of a past event can reach far beyond what other participants had ever intended. The shaping of self continues in the mind of the man or woman who relives, and reevaluates, the earlier event. In short, the event haunts this person because of the inner conversation he or she has with self about self (cf. Mead 1934; Strauss 1964). If redefining self and feeling occurs, the person may then create guidelines to avoid being cast into a surreal swirl of events over which he or she has no control.

Significant events also become important sources of comparison and contrast for self. Someone may accept the negative reflections of self given in the past event as to whom he or she was *then*, but not of the self of the present and future. Here, a significant event loses emotional power and subsequently becomes defined as a marker of the past, rather than a determining force in the present and future.

9

The Self in Time

Moment to moment. . . . That is the most comfortable way of living and the only way for me. There are times I move away from that and I get lost, but, by and large, I come back to that. It just seems to be the simplest, the least wear and tear. I mean it's like spending a whole bunch of time in the past or future just wears *me out, because the future is such an unknown that taking it pretty much as it comes up— I mean it's like I do make some plans but I find that that takes my energy from taking care of what's going on now. You can't give fully to what's going on now.*

I asked, "and the past?"

The past is nice to visit once in awhile. It's sort of—I can go back and get nurtured when I visit the past, mostly. *I mean there are some pretty nasty spots in the past, too, but by and large, it's nurturing stuff that I remember anyway. So, we remember the good stuff; we don't remember the bad stuff.*

Moving from moment to moment. Being in the moment. Trying to keep past and future from consuming him. Mark Reinertsen, at thirty-seven, has long attempted to be in the present. His renal failure and numerous debilitating complications span fourteen years. During the past five years, he had to cope with the deaths of the aunt and uncle who raised him, the loss of a lover, and the rigors of graduate school. Though Mark made schedules and his plans looked to the future, his self-concept remained in the present. By being in the present, he felt that he focused upon immediate events and intensified his involvement in them. Otherwise, his illness with its spiraling complica-

228

tions could overwhelm and devour him, leaving little of his preferred self intact.

Mark's self-concept became tied to the present; he saw and experienced himself as real, i.e., authentic, when he lived in the present. For him, leaving the past alone allowed him to attend to the present and enabled him to make his real, or fundamental, self an actual self. Being in the past jarred his real self, for he felt pressured to keep his thoughts, feelings, and actions—and therefore his self-concept—in the present.

Experiencing chronic illness may result in ill people's self-concepts becoming tied to the past, present, or future. Thus, time plays a central, albeit hidden, role in shaping self-concept. A once certain self-concept can become elusive and may shift and change through time, like a kaleidoscope that recombines and restructures pieces of the past, present, and future. New events result in recombining past, present, and projected future selves in different, shifting ways.

All the ways of experiencing time that I have described throughout the book influence locating the self in a particular timeframe. A questionable future can prompt people who anchored themselves to the future to seek a valued self in the present. When dull days replace vibrant years, the past can offer solace and refuge. Being disrupted by illness can spur the ill person to look beyond the present and locate the self in a brighter future.

How are chronically ill people's self-concepts imbedded in timeframes of past, present, and future? In which ways do time structures and time perspectives foster tying the self to a specific timeframe? Under which conditions do ill people's real selves become situated in specific timeframes? When do they view their experiences as revealing aspects of their past, present, or future real selves? How might prior timeframes for locating the self-concept change or continue?

An irretrievable past, an unsettling present, and an irrevocably changed future alter an individual's views of self. These altered views reflect shifts in the relatively stable foundation of the self-concept; the structure of it changes.

Significant events and turning points produce images of self that illuminate the direction and content of the emerging self.

Living one day at a time forces a once future-oriented person to think of self in relation to time differently. Although they do so in often invisible or implicit ways, people identify with some periods of time, events, and experiences but not with others. And their ways of viewing and relating to time affect their emerging selves. Select times, events, and experiences then become anchored to the self. In short the self is situated in time as well as in relationships.

To date, sociologists have largely viewed the self-concept as imbedded in and emerging from relationships. Granted, relationships are pivotal and influence a person's emerging self-concept. Yet those relationships develop during specific periods in a person's life, which may be circumscribed and time-limited. Family, friends, health professionals, and helpers observe, share, contribute to or create key events or periods of time in an ill person's life. Relationships not only exist within social structures, they exist within socially constructed times.

Goffman (1959), Turner (1976), Turner and Gordon (1981), and more recently, Denzin (1984; 1986) all point a way to studying what people take as their real selves. Turner argues that people do not view all their behaviors, attributes, or actions as reflecting their real selves (see Chapter 2 endnote 2). For Turner, the self consists of a relatively stable, organized core of qualities beyond self-esteem or idealized self-images through which people define and locate themselves. As such, this core of qualities becomes an object that does not simply replicate all that one does, says, or feels. Hence, the self-concept provides meanings that people attribute to themselves and unifies subjective experience over time (Charmaz 1981; Denzin 1986; Turner 1976).

Clearly, not all events, actions, periods of time, or even attributes, stick to and meld with self. But some do. I explore both the coercive conditions and autonomous choices that foster melding the self to a particular time frame. Further, ill people's self-concepts may shift their locations in the past, present, or future at different points in their illnesses. For example, a person who has been tied to the past or future may come to live in the present and to see self as situated within it.

Melbin (1987) argues that time is a container for activities and events. In an analogous way, time serves as a container for situating the self, although both process and product remain implicit. Assumptions about time lead people to act as if the past, present, and future were containers, or timeframes, that bounded their self-concepts. I treat these timeframes as largely analytically distinct for clarity, although, typically, they are experientially mixed. Though some people locate themselves rather firmly in the past, present, or future, they also experience a past, present, and future sliding together and must attend to these other timeframes, in whatever way they conceive them. I note this fluidity of time to avoid freezing people in one timeframe.

The Self in the Past

The past serves as a timeframe to contain varied events and to reflect diverse selves. Whether people slip into locating themselves in the past or actively seek to tie themselves to it depends upon the form of the past that they have experienced and remember. Thus, to discover how and why people come to situate their self-concepts in the past necessitates looking at their meanings about the past. What forms does the past take?

The Past as a Tangled Web

When people view their past as tangled, they try to locate themselves in the actions and events that formed it. They feel caught and overwhelmed by their past. They seek to *explain* and *account* for the events of the past that have brought them into the present (Lopata 1986). As one elderly man reflected, "I live in the past too much; I keep trying to figure out what happened." Living in the past pulls people into it—steadily—stealthily without their full awareness. They wonder if they contributed to past events. If so, they seek more than understanding these events. They feel compelled to come to some resolution or decision about them. Questions and feelings about individual responsibility tie people to the past. "How did it all happen?" "Did I do it to myself?" "Could I have handled my illness better?" "What if I had had less stress?" "What if I had known my diagnosis earlier?"

Here, the "what if's?" dive into the *past*, rather than leap into the future. By asking such questions, ill people begin to unravel their past. They study the past to understand and explain their present and to predict their future.

An overriding reason for striving to understand one's past is to avoid repeating it. In this case, the "what if's?" about the past lead directly to the future. "What if I caused it? Then I can change me and get healthier." Past and future loom large. The present narrows and feels tenuous. Being catapulted from a minor disability to total paralysis left Harriet Binetti dazed and bewildered. She studied the past because she questioned why her condition worsened so rapidly. She felt caught in a web of the past. Eight years later, she still asked, "How did it happen? Did the divorce trigger it?" She observed that before her divorce:

> When I'd have flare-ups and all, I always just came back from it, you know, pretty well . . . and even when I had problems, there was somebody who took care of everything. . . . When I got my divorce, within six months, I had a cane and I had two bad flare-ups . . . everything was on my shoulders, as far as the checkbook and all and, I don't know, I guess being alone. Being alone as far as security, I'm speaking. And it was just a lot for me to handle. Susan [her daughter] was fifteen then. Robert [her son] used to run away.

Harriet Binetti also studied the past to search for ways to avoid her earlier fate—nursing home placement. Most of her lump-sum divorce settlement went to a lawyer to defend her son against criminal charges. When she had no money, she had no choice in living arrangements. Harriet had struggled to survive in the three nursing homes through which she was shuffled. She looked back at those struggles in dread that she might face them again. Her fear of being put in another nursing home intensified when she thought of her frail, elderly mother, who might be relegated to a similar fate. For Harriet, a nursing home symbolized her worst possible future. She tried to live one day at a time, but her fears of having to relive her past pulled her back into that past. She attempted to disentangle certain strands of her past and tried to cut others that might ensnare her again. But paradoxically, her efforts kept her tied to the past.

The Familiar Past and Inexplicable Present

The past feels familiar when it is predictable, understandable, and close to self. This past does not require sorting; it seems self-evident. People allude to a familiar past most often when that past was unencumbered by illness. However, as I have suggested, a past *in* illness can also take on familiarity and predictablity.

Locating oneself in the past occurs when 1) people sense a radical disjuncture between a familiar past and the seemingly inexplicable or alien present, and 2) the self revealed in the present is untenable or unacceptable. These people feel the changes. Telling signs remind them. Numerous people noted declining mental faculties and failing bodies. Certainly, alcoholism, memory loss, and medication side-effects can make the present inexplicable and the past, by contrast, both comprehensible and comfortable (Feil 1985). But so can loneliness, depression, and exhaustion. In the aftermath of her stroke, May Sarton writes: "And [before] I felt so safe and well. Now I've been knocked down—and that is what is difficult—to be suddenly old. . . . A radical change of life" (1988:44). Under such conditions, people feel trapped in an alien present while their self-concepts reside in a familiar past. Sarton also comments, "I feel so cut off from what was once a self" (1988:97).

When the present marks a radical change, the past provides more than the security of familiarity, it offers a foundation for reconstructing an altered, if diminished, self-concept. In this sense, situating the self in the past can help one adapt to the present and shape a future. Taking strength from the past assuages fear, reduces shock, and overcomes disappointment. As a middle-aged man reflected:

There's a past that you remember and there's a past that's reality. Then there's a past that's—that's as much reality as ah, oh [searching for words], how could you say that? Remember seeing a scene, or a moment from childhood, for instance, that is particularly poignant. I guess I'm sure everyone has you know, memories, pictures or something. They're more than pictures, they're *feelings* and they're places to which you orient yourself in your life. And when, when you think about it, you think, you just think, who am I? What are my values? And those are the kind of places you go back to to reground yourself.

Locating oneself in the familiar past can take other forms. As I imply in Chapter 4, insulating self in illness routines can result in continuing to locate self in a past illness should health vastly improve (cf. Sacks 1984). In contrast, when the past illness evokes terror, people may remain in it without embracing sickness itself. Here, the past takes on an ominous, but unshakable, familiarity. Further, the present seems uncertain and unfathomable when doubts arise about a lasting recovery or about having a future at all. For example, Joanne Dhakzak's images of herself remained tied to her past with Hodgkin's lymphoma: "I'm too much in the past; I don't let myself move on and really create a life. It's like if I do anything important, I may lose it because the cancer might come back. So I don't let myself do anything; I don't give my life direction. You can waste life going through life like that."

Though her interests led toward pursuing a professional degree, she wondered if just making the commitment to attend graduate school would hasten another episode. She also worried that the stress of school and a job might make her sick again. Her feelings of being stuck in a dark past increased when she compared her life with her husband who sped into a bright future with his blossoming career. Meanwhile, her self-concept remained situated in a gnawing, frightening past, in which she felt inextricably trapped.

The Reconstructed Past

The reconstructed past, in contrast, typically shines bright with happiness, fullness, and vibrancy when viewed against the lived present. Here, ill people reject being identified by their lived present. Subsequently, they see their preferred selves within their reconstructed memories and begin to locate themselves in the past. As Maines, Sugrue, and Katovich (1983) observe, present realities shape what people remember. Recollections of possessing much greater vitality and, moreover, *validity* spur reconstructing and reliving the past. The comparative value of a past self further increases when a dark or empty future looms ahead. In short, a past self takes on fresh and expanded meaning when reconstructed and observed from the vantage point of the present. When actually experienced, however, the past may not have held such august meanings. But comparisons of past and present self make the former self seem unquestionably preferable.

Isolation and immersion in illness routines can foster situating oneself in the past because the present may lack a sense of being really lived. In this situation, it is almost as if people observe rather than live their own lives. For people who had predicated their self-concepts on action and productivity, time stands still, and the present offers scant material for constructing a valued self. For them, the present provides a distorted mirror of their real selves, since it only reveals shadows of their past selves. The present is grim, the future depressing. Therefore, they search their pasts for more valued selves.

Living in the past can lead to anchoring the self to it. Isolation, compounded by illness and confinement, can pull anyone into the past. Although eight months earlier, Heather Robbins had situated herself in the future, she now moved toward the past. Caring for her new baby kept her confined and separated from her earlier pursuits. She said, "Sometimes I see myself wanting to do things, but right now, I see myself being stagnant, and it's okay. So it's okay. And maybe that's why I've been living in the past right now, or I think a lot about the past. Because six months ago I wasn't. I was thinking about what I can do, not what I've done, and lately it's been thinking about what I've done. I realize I'm going to change." Unless restricted by illness, Heather Robbins will change because she is young. But those elders who lose a sense of evolving and endure poverty and confinement seldom have opportunities or encouragement to change. They remain in the past.

Locating the self in the reconstructed past turns on three major properties of immersion in illness: loss, unchanging time, and social isolation. Losses can encompass a lack of control over circumstances, choices, and self-definition, as well as health. Hence, people shake or mute these effects by anchoring themselves to images of a past self. For example, one man who lost agility and speech attempted to counter present images of self by informing others about his past accomplishments.

Experiencing unchanging time while immersed in illness, with its attendant constricted space and limited action, leads to a slowed time sense. The self contracts. Oliver Sacks relates his experience of hospitalization:

> I had no sense, no realization, of how contracted I was, how insensibly I had become contracted to the locus of my sickbed and sickroom—contracted in the most literal, physiological terms, but contracted too, in imagination and feeling. I had become a pygmy, a prisoner, an inmate—a patient—without the faintest awareness. We speak, glibly, of "institutionalization," without the smallest sense of what is involved—how insidious, and universal, is the contraction in all realms (not least the moral realm), and how swiftly it can happen to anyone, oneself. . . . Now I realized, such regression was universal. It would occur with any immobilization, illness or confinement. It was an unavoidable, natural shrinking down of existence, made bearable and untreatable because not realizable—not directly realizable. How could one know that one had shrunk, if one's frame of reference had itself shrunk? (1984: 156–157)

Consistent with Sacks, as space shrinks, days contract. Time narrows to the routines and rhythms of a hospital or household. With which qualities of lived time can these ill people construct a self? Because our society values action over reflection, would they not therefore look to past events in which they had been vital actors, or could appear to be so? For example, having to spend her last years in an institution shocked an eighty-five-year-old woman. She savored recounting stories about the days when she worked on the family ranch. By doing so, she salvaged and preserved a sense of the independence and diligence that earlier identified her. Despite being isolated, dependent, and frail, reclaiming and talking about her past self brought it into the present. Simultaneously, by valuing her past self, she gained strength to handle her present circumstances.

Thus, over months and years, people may tacitly come to form their present self-images from the past. A new resident in a board and care home described her counterparts as living in the past, "The past is all they talk about." Perhaps the past was all they had. →Statement about family environment / Support

Ill people can remain tied to another time, another era, that others may neither remember nor value. Further, if their health precludes projects, pursuits, and purposes with others beyond their daily care, they lose possibilities for projecting a shared present and future.[1] Their range of "possible selves" also contracts (Nurius 1989).

As lines between past and present blur, they seem to merge. Older ill people, particularly, sometimes speak of events as if they happened yesterday, when, in fact, they happened decades ago. This blurred time and collapsed chronology also foster developing a self in the past.

Having a self in the past is most visible when ill people judge the present, in general, and their present identities, in particular, by the *criteria* of the *past*. Without validation of that criteria, a self situated in the past becomes even more discernible. In short, the extent to which someone situates his or her self in the past becomes apparent through interaction.

Situating the self in the reconstructed past influences others' images of the person. Living a constricted life for years makes anyone seem a little "out of step," if not entirely a relic of the past, even when young. An ill person may be dimly aware of not being quite "in tune" with the times or "in touch" with events. Most likely, such individuals will not share the values and perspectives of those who "keep up with the times."

As times and ideas change, and ill people are systematically left out, the disparity increases between their situated selves and external events. Even so, someone might locate his or her self in the past for public display while simultaneously maintaining a self in the present that fits a narrowed life (cf. McMahan and Rhudick 1964; Revere and Tobin 1980–1981; Tarman 1988). For example, an educated and articulate elderly man who had lost his health, his family, and his money, was forced to spend his last years in an institution that served the poor. He regaled the residents, staff, and visitors with tales of his past political intrigues, powerful friends, and sexual adventures. He claimed a past self imbedded in regional circles of power and demanded deference due to his past associations and accomplishments. His tales underscored his past significance and laid claims for continued validation as the residents' unofficial spokesman.[2] His commanding voice and authoritative manner disallowed challenge to his claims.

This man used images of a past to construct a preferred self in the present. As Hendricks (1982) implies, having intentions lends a sense of continuity to time. Grasping the past and making it continuous with the present mutes and lessens the diminishment of self brought about by illness.

Parallels can be found in the "senile" aged. Naomi Feil argues that disoriented patients actually choose to retreat into the past. In her story of Mrs. Wohl, who worked for an electric company for fifty-eight years as a file-clerk and bookkeeper, Feil writes:

> That life is with her now as much as ever. Being a good worker is her reason for existence. Her purse is her file cabinet. She explains, "It's a measure for keeping time, not so much a pocketbook."
> Mrs. Wohl no longer moves in chronological clock-time. She tells time by how she feels. When we discuss time-change and her need to travel back to the past, she smiles, "I can travel anywhere I like. The company will pay the fare." (1985:94)

Even well-oriented ill people find that the self they recreate from the past remains fundamentally problematic. They no longer can confirm it with actions and relationships given in the present. Indeed, memory alone becomes the ultimate validation of this self, which leaves it fragile and tentative.

Despite occasionally finding an appreciative audience for his tales of the past, another elderly man could not turn them into a valued self in the present. His repetitious stories rambled and, frequently, bored his listeners. Also, he neither sparingly selected nor artfully timed his tales to support his present claims. As a result, others usually treated his stories as an old man's quaint relics to be noted, then disregarded.

Subsequently, such people may also question their value. Of course, the prior selves of many older ill people are wholly unknown, or unacknowledged by others, who, in turn, fail to act properly toward them. Instead, others' actions imply their negative assessments. And, in turn, these elders wish to reject, hide, or transcend a devalued identity. In short, the self given in the present situation is probably neither socially nor personally valued.

Last, though ill people may try to situate their self-concepts in the past, present concerns and future worries can intrude upon them. The weight of the present and future can disrupt their reverie and cut through their images of past selves. Then, they may view, and even affirm, the self that other people see as given in their present situation. Even people who anchor themselves the most in the past may attend to the present and future. An elderly man lived in a board and care residence and sustained himself with his many stories of his good deeds, now long past. His caretakers identified him as someone who lived in the past. Nevertheless, he, too, wondered about his future. After telling his tales over and over, he ended each interview with the haunting question, "Tell me, do you think I will ever get out on my own again?"

The Self in the Present

The self in the present is anchored to the here and now. Thereby time horizons stay close and neither past nor future assumes priority. When people make living one day at a time a habit, they come to anchor themselves to the present. Yet others also live in the present but remain relatively unaware of time or of self; they take for granted a self situated in the present.

Situating one's self in the present necessitates living in the present. How do people come to anchor their self-concepts to the present? When do they do it? What does it mean to them? Experiencing illness can affirm or accelerate lessons about living in the present gained from other experiences, such as self-exploration or therapy. A professor of dentistry had learned to reduce stress while in psychotherapy. He now advocated "not trying to carry the weight of the world" himself. He discovered that this stance also kept him in the here and now.

Fulfilling cherished goals permits someone to loosen bonds to the future. When an individual feels a sense of completion, striving toward the future and situating self within it can lessen. Earlier a middle-aged man had described himself as situated in the future. One year later, he said, "I feel like I'm more in the present. . . . Well, maybe I was hoping I would win an award. And I won one. . . . I don't seem to have as much time to think about the future, too; that's part of it. And the family relationships seem better now; they seem calmer and more constant. . . . Also I've gotten to do more things I wanted to do. I wanted to travel for years and I finally did it."

Experiencing earlier losses can set the stage for learning to live in the present. A spouse's death, an adult child's disability, a forced retirement, or an unanticipated divorce can cause someone to begin to live in the present. When I asked Nancy Swenson what had helped her to learn to live in the present, she said, "The *illness*. I think it's a big—I think it was the thought maybe I'm not going to be here and I should start enjoying things and, and counseling. . . . [Earlier] my house burned down and I lost everything. And then my stepdaughter ripped off all of my good jewelry . . . [that] always meant a lot to me."

Nancy Swenson had already lost many symbols of her past—photographs, clothes, furniture, mementos, even her income tax records. Shortly thereafter her marriage crumbled. Her losses separated her from her past and the symbols of it. Then illness and possible death destroyed her future plans and drew her into the present.

Reinterpreting earlier goals and pursuits as unimportant makes it possible to relinquish them. The professor of dentistry reflected, "I spend a lot less time agitating myself about school politics. There are many things about the dental school that bother me. . . . I have fought and argued and held out against graduating students that everybody else said you've got to graduate and so on. And when they did graduate, they passed the boards like nothing. . . . Who knows whether you are right or wrong? And so why waste that wonderful energy on something that's rather less than beautiful?"

Valuing immediately realizable goals makes the present livable (Jones 1988). When people try to live one day at a time, they set only immediate goals. Later, they may learn to set some future goals without wedding themselves to them. For example, Lois Jaffe observes, "People ask me if I plan for the future. . . . Yes, I plan for the future—but only with my head. My heart and my soul are in the present, in what I'm doing today" (1977:208).

Learning to live in the present reflects a specific form of the present. I turn next to consider three forms of the present. The number, pacing, and quality of events contained in each form distinguishes them. Different definitions of succession and duration within these forms of the present shape meanings of it (Flaherty 1987; Fraisse 1984; McGrath and Kelley 1986).[3]

The Filled Present

→ sounds like behavior of depressed, coping behaviors

Situating the self in the filled present means anchoring the self to a present crammed with activities and events. Activity and speed distinguish the filled present, rather than emotional involvement. A sense of rapid succession of present events validates the self. When people live in a present so filled with activities and medical regimens, they make comments like, "I don't have time for the pain."

Some people pack the present by squeezing many experiences, activities, and events into short spaces of time. As a result, they do more than their healthier counterparts (Charmaz 1987). They try to take control of themselves and their lives, despite illness. Of course, they may take risks with their health. They may not attend to developing symptoms or problems because their busy lives so involve them. Vera Mueller once described herself as turning blue, experiencing chest pain, and having an irregular heart beat. However, she did not keep her doctor's appointment. She commented, "I didn't have time to go over there [to the doctor's office]. . . . I was busy writing a paper, and I didn't want to be interrupted."

Cramming one's days can reflect either a lifelong pattern or an awareness of a foreshortened life. These men and women reason that they must pursue their interests and potential now, for they might not have another chance. When Mark Reinertsen believed that he would not live past thirty, he filled his days, quickened the pace of his activities, and crammed in as many events as possible. He also resolved "to let the past go," without dwelling on it or on the future. After doing so, he began to anchor himself to the present. In an interview eight years ago, he noted the change: "I'm in the here and now a lot more. But there was a time in my life when I wasn't in the here and now, and now I am most of the time rather than being back there or up there. It doesn't do any good. I can't do anything about back there and I can't do anything about up there. So, why be there?"

Mark Reinertsen believed that his earlier ruminations about the past had prevented him from handling the present and from knowing himself within it. His present self emerged from past selves (Mead 1934). Though he sensed continuity of self with the past, he guarded against having the past cloud the present. Similarly, he resisted having a tenuous future blight it.

Later, Mark moved from a filled present to an intense present. His story suggests how people change the timeframe of their situated selves. Earlier, while on dialysis, his future had looked precarious, limited, and foreshortened. Two years later, he saw his transplant as a reprieve. At this point, he reduced his activities considerably, but involved himself more deeply in those he kept. Although his physical condition necessitated this reduction, his life gained meaning and intensity. He felt that he could hope for a future. He began to experience an intense, though slow, present. Subsequently, he savored the present and enjoyed small pleasures such as petting his cat or sitting quietly and listening to music, pastimes that his packed days had precluded. In short, when he could see a future ahead of him, he moved into an intense present.

The Slowed-down Present

Scaling down the present by reducing the timing, pacing, number, and intensity of involvements fosters anchoring the real self to the present. Like the filled present, activity and speed also distinguish the slowed present, but in reverse. In contrast, the slowed down present may be driven by feelings. When choices dwindle and sorrow increases, the slowed down present seems to expand; time moves slowly and seems empty (cf. Aaronson 1972). As one man said, time is "spaces to fill between periods of sleep." May Morganson said, "I don't do much; my life is very boring."

However, when people can *choose* to live in a slowed down present, like taking one day at a time, they feel they have more control over the present and more readily attach themselves to it. As evident in preceding chapters, experiencing a slowed down present can occur without situating the self within it.

Accepting a slowed down present does not come easily, and these men and women often wished to return to more active lives. For example, Ann Rorty remarked:

> I think sometimes when I feel good . . . of—when a few hours a day, or a day where, you know, where everything is kind of mellowed out and even though I'm still having a little bit of pain, I'm thinking, "Well, you know, maybe I could do it . . . maybe I could get back there and . . ." and then I'll go do something and the pain shoots, you know, through my hips or down my legs. . . . And then I go, "No, I don't think I'm ready yet." You know, I don't think I'm ready to tackle it yet, because I know what I would have to do. Like on my last job—I couldn't do it. I know I couldn't do it. So that kind of flies out the window.

Depression, disability, medications, and mental dysfunction can all contribute to slowing down. A middle-aged man said, "My head is still just, you know, reeling and I don't know whether it's from lack of oxygen . . . but in terms of functioning and doing stuff that I used to do . . . I may not be able to do that again."

In the meantime, this man looked at the bright side by taking time for reflection. He remarked:

> This is a very rare opportunity you have to sit and look at things and from a state of quietness, [after] a state of getting caught up in this rat race that we all make for ourselves. . . . This is the chance to kind of sit back and see what it's all about and see where the values really lie in your life. . . . It doesn't make any difference to move unless you have someplace to move to. And you know, unless you assess what things are meaningful to you, how do you know which things you want to come out and grow and what things you don't?

This man had some choice as to how to relate to time and perhaps, might be able to redirect himself. In contrast, for many residents of institutions, the slowed down present is endless. They are assigned to their placements and become resigned to their fates. These residents may anchor their self-concepts only to select events, especially those in which their anonymity fades. At visiting time, these lonely people station themselves in the front lobby to converse with anyone passing by. Hungry for compassion, for contact, for connection with the "real world," they grab a visitor's hand and hope for a momentary pause. A frequent visitor remarked, "They say, 'Oh, it's been so long since you've been here,' and it's only been a week!"

Some residents anchor themselves to their times with regular visitors. Upon escorting me to my car, a sixty-two-year-old resident of a board and care home said to me, "You asked what time meant to me. Only times like when that little girl [sic] [his thirty-one-year-old volunteer] comes to take me out or you visit mean anything. All the rest means nothing. *Nothing*."

For these residents, moments of acknowledgment and acceptance light their slowed present and shine meaning upon it. Though bright, like a spray of fireworks against a dark sky, such moments may be almost as evanescent.

The slowed down present can take a heavy toll on people whose hopes, dreams, and plans were predicated on activity and intensity. Should a person maintain an earlier criteria for self-worth, anger, frustration, and blame follow. Bursts of anger give voice to enormous frustration and disappointment. Furious blame gets hurled, like arrows, at doctors, nurses, and spouses.

Anger and blame are ready means for enlivening a slowed down present and for bringing intensity into the day. People who use these means resist linking their self-concepts to the slowed down present. Nonetheless, the passing days can grind and deplete their spirits. Once directed outward, anger, frustration, and blame now cut inward. When others' judgments reinforce and magnify these people's self-blame, they become further locked into their slowed down present. "Why don't you go back to work?" "If you just had a better attitude, you'd get better."

Here, accepting a self in the slowed down present requires changed expectations of self and criteria for self-worth. Simply maintaining a "positive" attitude and warding off depression can become the criteria for a valued self. While immersed in illness, Bonnie Presley still aspired to become a painter. She told herself, "I could change those [negative] thoughts to be positive. . . . Don't have negative feelings; don't express negative emotion; use that energy into something else. . . . I want to take this energy that I have and that anger, because I'm sick, and put it there into my work. If that's possible."

A focus on illness and regimen fosters ill individuals' accepting a slowed down pace and keeping their real selves in the present. As time passes, a slowed down pace may come to feel secure and offer a foundation for ill people's real selves.

The Intense Present

The self in the intense present emerges from the type and quality of events in the present. A sense of passion, authenticity, and involvement distinguishes the intense present. To ill people, present events have force; they cast their lives into new forms with new concerns, and seemingly sweep them into the here and now. The present feels fully lived (Denzin 1984; Flaherty 1987). The past separates from the present and the future grows distant.

Any reflective individual may experience an intense present

while ill, especially in the immediacy and urgency of critical illness. Locating one's self-concept within that present, however, goes beyond merely experiencing intensity; it means tying vivid feelings and passionate convictions to the self. Then, people try to perpetuate and to live within the force, urgency, and clarity of the intense present, as they anchor their self-concepts to it. Writer Susan Sontag captured that intensity when interviewed about having cancer. She said:

> It [thinking about death] has added a fierce intensity to my life and that's been pleasurable.
>
> It sounds very banal, but having cancer does put things into perspective. It's fantastic knowing you're going to die; it really makes having priorities and trying to follow them very real to you. (*San Francisco Chronicle* 1978)

A renewed vitality of spirit and purpose marks and radiates a vivid present, despite, perhaps, diminished physical vigor. For example, Nancy Swenson described her present self and life as having far more depth than in the past. She added, "But I am definitely on a decline, a lot of things . . . that were no problem before, I mean even a year ago . . . I used to love to mow my lawn . . . and now I find it's such an effort; it's such an effort."

These men and women throw themselves into selected pursuits, which range from the grand to the mundane—from writing an autobiography to living simply but independently. With the intense present comes a sense of urgency—urgency to act, to experience, and to bond with other people. Vera Mueller described her sense of urgency as "taking today as it's presented to me and using it, making the absolute most of it." Similarly other people feel a sense of urgency to finish projects, to appreciate what they had taken for granted, to affirm attachments, and to right conflicted relationships.

The self in the intense present develops when ill people 1) can look forward to a "normal" life again due to recovery or marked improvement, 2) have faced and accepted death, and 3) have reviewed and reevaluated their lives. Believing that one has recovered or markedly improved often leads to feeling intensely alive, even resurrected. A man who had an angioplasty

what does this mean ??

remarked, "I felt like a million dollars. I was bright; I felt more energetic, more alive—I just—it was an amazing thing. . . . And it [his cardiac rehabilitation program] has made, as far as I am concerned, a new man of me."

After a young woman with diabetes adopted a more precise method of monitoring her blood sugar levels, she said, "I feel so much better now; the difference is amazing. My husband said, 'You're like your old self again—like you were before the diabetes.' I feel like so much more is possible for me now. I feel like I'm living each moment now."

These people feel that they have had a reprieve, a new opportunity to make an ideal self real. Their real self is a survived self. With the ordeal just behind them, they view their lives as having new possibilities, fresh starts, and added opportunities. They feel invigorated physically and therefore, perhaps, attend more closely to the present.

Unlike people who gain intensity by accepting death, these individuals may feel victorious over illness and death. In their view, they fought illness, defeated it, and left it behind. The present expands as a future becomes possible. Previously, they may have lived one day at a time to keep death and debility at bay. But their present remained limited, circumscribed in intensity and meaning, as well as in length.

In contrast, believing, as Susan Sontag did, that one has faced and accepted illness and death also leads to situating the self in the intense present. The certainty of one's mortality—and its imminence—casts a vivid light on the present. Nancy Swenson remarked, "Isn't it a shame that it takes illness for someone to realize what's important in life?" A woman with breast cancer told journalist Susan Schwartz, "If you face death, life becomes more valuable. I had never been really here, in the present, before. I always looked ahead or worried about the past. Now, I feel like I'm really here. I'm sorry that I had to learn the hard way [by having cancer]" (1979:1b).

Here, the real self in the intense present is an ill self—illness becomes part of self. Illness may even form the foundation of the self and self-value. And illness may provide constant reminders of limited time. After his life-saving surgery, a middle-aged man reflected:

248 ILLNESS, THE SELF, AND TIME

But having been through that, the thing that impresses me the most and is the most important for me to keep real clear is the volatileness of life. And what do you do then? . . . It's like there's no point to spend all that time worrying about all that stuff [work, deadlines, status]; it's like building sandcastles. If you're on the beach, that's a good thing to do, but don't get upset when they fall down, because that's what they are going to do. The clearer you are on that, the less stressed out you are going to get when you build your sandcastle and the corner crumples off, or a wave comes in because that's the nature of it. So then it kind of refocuses . . . my view of what I'm doing here and what's meaningful about it and what isn't.

Living in the intense present fosters awareness of elapsing time. Vera Mueller made this contrast; "In the back of my head, there was always I'll have tomorrow to fix what I didn't fix today. . . . Well, my life is the reverse of that now. Don't put off what you can take care of today."

These people often reorder time to realize their priorities. Vera elaborated: "Once the day is over, you can't go back and do it again. It is gone *forever*. It's a once-in-a-lifetime opportunity and so time has gotten very critical for me. *Every single day* is a brand new opportunity to realize who I am and to be who I want to be. And any moment that is wasted by not striving toward realizing that potential is a moment lost forever."

Although Vera Mueller had already redirected her life before her sister's untimely death, this significant event brought her into the intense present. She said:

I know what I want to accomplish before I die. That's all very sudden following Cynthia's death. . . . When they put me in my grave, what I want people to be thinking about and feeling and reminiscing about is the fact that, "Yeah, the first few years of her life were pretty fucked up, but she got her head together; she found what she wanted to do and she did it, and she did it with all the exuberance and, you know, happiness and eagerness for life that anybody could possibly want." I want my children to be able to think back, "Yeah, Mom lived her life, by gosh. Mom enjoyed living." I want that to be the legacy I leave behind. I don't want to leave them with the legacy that my parents, my mother and my father and my sister left me, which is one of feeling that their lives were wasted tragedies.

Situating the self in the intense present tends to be a fragile arrangement. Like the glow of compassion during religious holidays or the commitment to New Year's resolutions, daily routines dull and supersede the intense present. The wonder of having a reprieve lessens. The excitement of dramatic improvement fades. The imminence of death gives way to mundane pursuits. Several months later, the young woman with diabetes said that her sense of an expanding self and a vivid present had faded, despite the new regimen. She added, "It's just a regimen, Kathy. It's a better regimen, but it is just a regimen." A year later, a man who had had bypass surgery forgot how precious time had been. Two years after her mastectomy, Susan Sontag said of the stark reality of facing death and following priorities, "That has somewhat receded now; . . . I don't feel the same urgency. In a way, I'm sorry; I would like to keep some of that feeling of crisis" (*San Francisco Chronicle* 1978). Five years later, Vera Mueller remarked that "the sense of urgency is gone, at least consciously." Though the present may lose a sense of vitality and intensity, ill people may continue to live in the present.

As ill people reorder their priorities and locate themselves in the present, they may find that rather than settling for less, they have gained more. Nancy Swenson stated, "I was always trying to achieve and strive for things. I was always looking to the future. All the things that I was looking to achieve, I found that they aren't important to me anymore."

Similarly, reappraisals of self result in efforts to change. Judgmental individuals become less so and acquiescent people become more autonomous. In both cases, they observe their lives more closely (Mann, Siegler, and Osmond 1972). As a result, people follow new pursuits and seek new friends. Nancy Swenson said, "You find much more meaningful people in your life."

The flip side of observing life closely is to focus inward on self to the extent that one sinks into it. But a more positive paradox occurs when people discover that they can face the future with more ease and look back on the past with less regret. Without the pressure of mapped futures, they can anticipate selected future events without feeling trapped by them. As one woman explained, "I look forward to them [future plans] but it's not like my life revolves around them." Similarly, by not clinging to the past, these people do not ruminate about lost chances. And a final paradox: by living in the present, these people believe they create better pasts. Nancy Swenson advised, "Whatever time it is, relish what you have of it because you can always savor it; it never goes away."

The Self in the Future

Promise or threat beckons people who situate their self-concepts in the future. Like fisherfolk who cast their lines in the sea, these people cast their self-concepts into the future along with their hopes and plans. They tie themselves to future plans, possibilities, and dreams.[4] Why they do so turns on whether their lives revolve around illness and whether their time perspective takes emphasizing the future for granted. Hence, tethering oneself to the future can take sharply different forms, and these forms can change at different points in people's lives.

Situating one's self-concept in the future means living in the future, directing one's thoughts, actions, and plans toward the future. Hence, the future, rather than the past or present, assumes distinct focus. Specific meanings of the future shape how ill people project themselves into it. In turn, how someone lives in the future shapes the self cast within it. In the following discussion, I address how people attach themselves to what they believe are positive futures: the completed self, the assumed self, and the immortal self. However, as I suggested earlier, immobilizing fears can also shackle someone to a dark future—dependency and death.

The Dreaded Future

By residing in a dreaded future, people can, albeit unwittingly, attach themselves to it for periods of time—long periods. Thus, they live in silent terror and wait—for months, years, even decades—for that future they know will come. Meanwhile, they study each developing symptom, each possible sign foreshadowing the dreaded future, the certain fate. The fear, dread, and terror *of* dependency and death can shape the meaning of this future, as well as actual dependency and dying.

These ill people view a sharply defined image of the future through a refracted lens and, therefore, make it clearer and bring it closer. To the extent that they narrow and intensify their focus on a dreaded future, its image increasingly magnifies and engulfs them. Life is out of control. These ill people disengage from the present. The past fades. They feel catapulted into inescapable doom.

Not surprisingly, feeling trapped by an uncontrollable future also traps one in a dialectic of negative emotions. Anger, self-pity, and depression lead to and strengthen the feeling of being trapped. In turn, feeling trapped magnifies and extends anger, self-pity, and depression. Though perhaps unspoken, definitions of an uncontrollable future circumscribe interaction. Thus, illness supersedes and dominates life, for illness bodes of death. Quite possibly, a time perspective entrenched in the future contributes to developing a trapped self in a dreaded future.

The Improved Future

Hoping or planning for a completed self means looking to the future for a fuller realization of self. People who do so desire or expect their future selves to realize present potentials, to expand understanding, and to fulfill goals. They often envision a preferred self in the future and pin their self-concepts to it. That preferred self may serve as a bridge between a real self in the actual present and an ideal self in a better future. A middle-aged man with diabetes described himself and his future this way:

I tend—tended, at least in recent years—to be a future-situated person, that things will get better. My wife and I will come to greater understanding and sympathy for one another and, in fact, that happened. I'll be more relaxed about my life. I'll remember that it isn't phony to be pleasant to people and, in fact, if I do that, the chances are that they'll be pleasant to me. Yes, so I guess there's a lot of self-improvement runs through me. My work will be better known—thinking about this time next year, and so forth; there's that.

Plans and projects encourage anchoring oneself in an improved future. After a turbulent first marriage, a young woman felt exhilarated about her plans to remarry and about her better prospects at work. She looked forward to a more stable and happier future; she saw her real self in the future. When I first interviewed her, Heather Robbins also anchored her self in the future. She said, "I've always dealt in the future. . . . And what I'm working for is not now; it's definitely not now, it would be later. So it's like everything we [she and her husband] do now is just temporary. It's a step to get somewhere."

Though Heather Robbins had already tied her self-concept to the future before she became ill, she found that she redirected her goals afterwards:

> Even with this disease, I think that I am a lot less handicapped than a lot of people who have all of their senses and their facilities . . . and can walk and can talk but can't see [what's significant]. That is another thing this disease gave me that I didn't have before. I had goals that were meant to be selfish goals to make money. . . . It didn't matter who got stepped on to get there, either, but that's just not the way it is anymore.

Not everyone who tied themselves to the future saw doing so as entirely good. Rather, their views, as well as their lives, led them into the future, despite their misgivings about it. The future tugs at these people, constantly pulling them into it. As the man above said:

> Of course, I've tried to live in the present just—that's what poets tell you to do, by and large, although they also tell you to remem-

ber the past. . . . Otherwise it [keeping oneself in the present] is an ideal, but not really a possibility for very long at a time. So I would like to answer that I live in the present, that's what I think a person should do. But I think from what friends have let me know, that I live in the future. I want to know what's coming next and where what I'm saying will lead me.

Thus, people saw themselves in the future when their thoughts, plans, and actions led them there.

Not all images of future self are easily disclosed. Several men and women revealed anchors to a future self that they could tell few people. Though one woman with multiple sclerosis managed the present and sometimes dreaded the future, part of her remained anchored to a future self unencumbered by illness. Simultaneously, she accepted the medical model and followed her neurologist's advice. Meanwhile, she rejected his statements that her disease was progressive and unamenable to reversal. Given her plight and her self-image as a realistic, responsible adult, she could not reveal her hope for the future. For her, the completed self meant a renewed body and spirit, the improved future meant recovered health.

The Taken-for-Granted Future

When people simply assume that their self-concepts are cast into the future, they readily situate themselves in it. For them, reality lies in the future. The past recedes quickly and may be forgotten. The present provides the path to the future. Hence, plans for the future shape the present and keep these people moving forward into the future.

Because these men and women take their stance for granted, they find the possibility that other individuals might not share it to be a bit startling. "Of course I see myself largely in the future, doesn't everyone? You've got to go forward." Time moves on an upward plane—progressive and better. A woman's disabilities from multiple sclerosis caused her to relinquish a job she loved and to give up driving, a passport out of confinement in her suburban town. Although her activities had become more curtailed and her days more isolated, she did not take refuge in the past. She said, "I'm living now in tomorrow. The past is past. I'm taking care of today and looking forward into tomorrow. I have a saying, 'You can't look backwards into the future.' " When I asked her what that meant to her, she said, "Well, why try to go back and undo the past? You can't go back and live in the past—let's live in the future."

For her, the future did not preclude further disability. She faced that. When I asked her how she defined the future, she said, "I see it as continuing my life until my husband retires, then doing what he wants to do. I don't see anything but forward and upward. In fact, if I get into a wheelchair, I'll go with him wherever they'll let me go."

Her stance preceded illness and reflected a lifelong time perspective. She observed, "I think generally I always looked ahead instead of to the past. I've never been one to live in the past. When bad things happen, that's fine, well let's go on. I think it was an indirect lesson from my dad."

Unlike people who could look ahead only if their bodies remained intact, this woman found her perspective useful to ward off depression and to move out of it. Thus, she tried to move on and avoid becoming stuck and down. She said, "You just feel like you've been dealt a bad deck of cards. You just figure why? I think, 'How down.' I pick myself up and go on."

Maintaining this perspective while facing adversity depends on having a reason to live and an enduring sense of self-worth. Hence, social support can smooth the path into the future.

Similar assumptions can link people to a future that disallows further illness and disability. A paradox develops. People who hold these assumptions make promising candidates for arduous regimens and rehabilitation programs. They will work hard, take their programs seriously, and struggle to achieve small gains. But they expect payoffs for their efforts—progressive improvement, recovered vitality, a better future. If these rewards do not materialize, their enthusiasm melts into anger and depression. After several hefty defeats, they lose their seeming resilience. They feel cheated, betrayed, and diminished. And then, they may abandon their hopes and take refuge in the past.

The Everlasting Future

Views of self and of the future shift when death feels imminent. Thus, people who once lived in the past or present may now tie themselves to what comes after death. The quest for immortality gives life meaning. Creating an immortal self means that one's life made a difference; it had a purpose. That purpose may take two directions: to provide tangible proof of one's value, and to free an encaged spirit.

Though some people tie their real selves to a religious or spiritual belief, others create an immortal self through their work and their products, and thereby preserve their identity (Lifton 1968; Unruh 1983). Hence, they may immortalize their real self in the future by collecting prized objects, by writing a book, recording their life history, or reminiscing with family about their roles in past dramas. In this way they create their "symbolic immortality" (Lifton 1968). They live on in the future by turning the minds and touching the hearts of those who follow them.

If people feel caged in the present, they may reach for the future. If they feel locked in to a failing body, a limited life, and a hopeless present (cf. West 1984), they may look beyond the future for release and relief. They want to die. If they believe in a hereafter, they feel that death gives them freedom and immortality. For them, reality resides in the future—beyond life as they now know it.

Ron Rosato felt crushed by his physical dependence and spiraling complications from multiple sclerosis. When he compared his views with those of the people in his multiple sclerosis support group, he also began to allude to his view of himself: "They carried on in reality and me knowing that this is not reality, I mean to experience this stuff, this is not reality. . . . The only things they explored were ways to be comfortable in wheelchairs and stuff like that. And I just couldn't relate to that. I mean there I was with this problem that was getting worse and worse and there was no cure. . . . I was looking for depth."

A severe infection had kept Ron in the hospital for several weeks. He had wished to die; instead, he recovered. He said:

I believed in God, some type of God, and I said, "Man, get me out of here! Get me out of this body. Accept my spirit." And, because my spirit needs to be free, you know. Didn't happen.

I don't think of death as gloomy; I see it as a release. I was wishing so *much* for it. And now it doesn't scare me at all, at all. But I wish and I wonder when it will happen. . . . I'm ready, I think.

When new purposes emerge, an individual may anchor the self in the future rather than the past. Goldie Johnson had tried to take refuge in the past when her health plummeted. After her near-death experience, she saw herself and her future differently:

I see myself in the future now. If you'd asked where I saw myself eight months ago, I would have said, "the past." I was so angry then because I had been so active. And to go downhill as fast as I did—I felt life had been awfully cruel to me. Now I see myself in the future because there's something the Lord wants me to do. Here I sit all crumpled in this chair not being able to do anything for myself and still there's a purpose for me to be here. [Laughs.] I wonder what it could be.

What does He want me to do?

10

Lessons from the Experience of Illness

What lessons does the foregoing journey into illness provide? To which dilemmas does it point? To conclude the book, I offer a brief reflection about the effects of illness upon the self. During this reflection, I also draw upon how lived time contributes to those effects. And in closing, I show how lessons from the experience of illness illuminate needed changes for social policy.

The effects of illness upon the *self* range from loss to transcendence (Charmaz 1983b; Denzin 1986). For most people, the effects of illness fall in between loss and transcendence—small victories for self, major comebacks to self (Charmaz 1973), repeated tests of self. Mostly, chronically ill people try to be themselves; they try to live with their illnesses, which I have dealt with throughout the book. The course of chronic illness results in physical losses, sometimes mental losses, frequent social, psychological, and economic losses. When do these losses translate into loss of self? How is it that some people can transcend such losses? I turn here to look at loss and transcendence of self directly.

Loss of self means being involuntarily dispossessed of former attributes and sentiments that comprise one's self-concept, as well as the actions and experiences upon which they are based. It also means losing the self-definitions with which one had most identified. With loss of self, earlier boundaries of the self-concept shrink and become permeable. The self grows vulnerable to demeaning images reflected by others. The attrition of former attributes and sentiments results in changed feelings about self. Resignation follows. Hence, loss of self results in passivity.

257

Transcendence of self means that the self is more than its body and much more than an illness. Thus, illness does not fill or flood the self, even though it may fill and flood experience. Transcendence implies self-acceptance, rather than any acceptance of illness cloaked in stigmatized images and expectations of resignation. In addition, transcendence implies reevaluation and renewal. Achieving transcendence requires making choices and taking action.

Both loss and transcendence emerge from the experience of illness and the respective meanings that people confer upon it. Yet loss and transcendence are not static states of being, for one individual may experience both—sometimes dramatically, although at different points in his or her illness. Further, distance in chronological time between loss and transcendence can shorten when relapses, complications, and crises are unrelenting. With each episode, another physical loss. With each event, another possibility for knowing self.

Loss and transcendence are grounded in time—in moments, in good days and bad days, and in lengthy durations of time. Moreover, loss and transcendence become products of lived time and reflect meanings of it.

Loss and transcendence can be elusive when the processes creating them remain implicit—particularly when the person is unfamiliar with the course of illness and the ways of medical care. Thus, the events that give rise to loss or transcendence of self can remain unnoted or normalized by ill people. Similarly, as I showed in Chapter 8, definition of the significance of an event or period of time may occur long after someone has actually experienced it. Thus, what proves to be a turning point may only become apparent in retrospect by noting contrasts. Hence, experiencing loss of self can be an insidious process. As such, occasional visitors may witness it more readily than the men and women who experience it.

Certainly not everyone gains transcendence. Experiencing loss after loss can produce numbness (Lifton 1968) and a shrinking of self. Transcendence is something of a fragile state, for affirming it may rely largely upon the person who experiences it. Further, ill people may feel that they have transcended their illnesses at certain points only to plummet into loss at other times. For example, diagnosis of another serious illness can rupture a hard-won sense of transcendence. Nevertheless, transcendence is possible if ill people have time for reflection, gain the tools to do it, and define essential qualities of self as distinct from their bodies. Encouragement from others to reflect and to define a valued self beyond a failing body supports transcendence. Moreover, others' acclaim of the ill person's perseverance, courage, or strength may prompt his or her definitions of transcendence. Suffering an onslaught of troubles without flinching often gives ill people a sense that they have faced the worst and have transcended it. Hence, transcendence may develop from suffering tremendous physical, psychological, and social losses.

Loss of self derives from how meanings of bodily and mental competence shade self-definition. It also derives from the social meanings and spiraling consequences of illness. Thus, loss of self occurs with the help other people—sometimes enormous amounts of such "help." In contrast, transcendence sometimes occurs despite other people. Furthermore, realizing transcendence can necessitate separating the self from symbols of productivity, accomplishment, and success held by society.

The struggle for control of self in illness is a struggle against loss and, sometimes, for transcendence. The devastating losses from illness are apparent in the preceding pages. But, as I suggest, the struggle against loss might remain implicit for months and years, and whatever transcendence is gained may only be realized in retrospect. For many people, the struggle against loss arises in their efforts to live as they had in the past and to fulfill their responsibilities as they see them in the present and future. If they can keep illness in the background of their lives, their physical losses may seem as imperceptible as aging but accrue just as steadily.

Whether people struggle against loss at all becomes evident when illness dominates their lives. If they struggle, they do so for control of the defining images of self, for control over their bodies, and sometimes, for control over death.

Relative loss and transcendence of self turn on autonomy. People can lose much, but retain a sense of a transcendent self when they believe that they still make autonomous choices despite vastly circumscribed possibilities, and when they can preserve or create self-respect. Certainly it helps if other people support choices and demonstrate respect, which fosters maintaining self-respect. The self-respect and autonomy inherent in transcendence reflect trust in oneself and in one's sense of internal and external realities.

Maintaining such trust in self often becomes problematic during the vicissitudes of a chronic illness. Experiencing illness can erode earlier trust in self. It can also nurture earlier self-doubts. Subsequently, autonomy withers from within and, likely, is stiffled from without. Loss of self in illness mirrors this loss of autonomy. Loss of autonomy undermines the actions, emotions, and beliefs upon which the self had been built. The loss of autonomy that accompanies erosion of trust in self usually occurs long before the person realizes it, just as someone may have attained transcendence before defining it.

Autonomy means constructing independent choices and actions based upon reasoning (Cassell 1983). Control, in contrast, may be taken for granted and tied to feeling.[1] Practical dilemmas for ill people often concern the boundaries of control. Voluntarily loosening or relinquishing control in certain areas to preserve autonomy in others can help ill people maintain and develop valued aspects of self. Then, the meanings gained through experiencing illness deepen the self and the sense of self-knowledge. Paradoxically then, through the experience of wrestling for control of defining images of self, and abandoning conventional symbols of control, ill people may gain autonomy.

For those people who gain a sense of autonomy, their stories of illness may shift from chronicles of loss to tales of transcendence. Subsequently, ill people may look back upon the past and reconstruct their timemarkers and turning points into chronologies of a changed, more aware self, which documents their development.

The struggle for control is a struggle to achieve balance. For many ill people, it is a struggle between controlling the illness and becoming controlled by it, and by extension, other people. In essence, ill people struggle to prevent illness from inundating their self-concepts. Their emphasis on control frequently reflects implicit assumptions about time and body drawn from the wider culture, such as trying to relate to clock-time only through conventionally prescribed ways or expecting one's body to function like everyone else's. Should ill people accept such beliefs, their beliefs turn against them as their illness and disability increase. If so, their assumptions about controlling their bodies, or at least their appearances, force them to retreat to invisible, isolated lives.

Thus, a struggle for control may not work. In a larger sense, experiencing chronic illness threatens to puncture widely held beliefs of the nature of individual control in contemporary society. These beliefs assume control not only over one's time and body, but also over one's self and fate. Diminished control, in turn, diminishes a self predicated on assumptions of free choice and immediate action, when control stands as the measure of self. When ill people have little control, they may use that which they do have in ways that confound those around them. Hence, their actions can easily be misinterpreted. For example, someone who avoids disclosure of illness may do so as a way of maintaining control. However, other people may interpret this avoidance as denial or manipulation.

What implications does studying the self in time have for the medical care system? The implications turn on how illness intersects with the person's life. Thus, the person's age and the defined degree of progression of the illness shape these implications. Studying the self in time does reveal how the system encourages the forgotten chronically ill, especially older people, to look to their pasts for self-worth since the system offers them only a meager present and a bleak future.

By looking at the self in time, we can observe the implications for the medical care system throughout the process of illness. The experience of ill people is often taken as a direct reflection of their position as patients within the medical care system. Under certain conditions, their position can render them powerless. But the picture is more complex. For months and years, many people with chronic illnesses lead lives largely apart from the system. During those periods of time, other identities than that of being a patient—or for that matter, being a person with a chronic illness—assume priority.

What happens to chronically ill people within the medical

care system is part of an emergent process, rather than the reflection of static positions. Contacts with the medical care system can come at crucial points in an ill person's life or at points that they later define as markers of a revised life course. As a result, health care professionals affect ill people's lives at significant times. Clearly, rude discoveries, demeaning messages, and shocking news can accrue during the course of medical care if practitioners undermine or negate ill people during negative identifying moments, identifying crises, and significant events. Should the negative definitions of self in those events stick, then the ill person's autonomy diminishes.

As evident in stories in preceding chapters, ill people may accept negative definitions of self initially, then struggle against them and reject them. This struggle not only leads them to reject the medical care professionals who made those negative definitions, but also, in many cases, their treatment recommendations. To the extent that ill people become embroiled in identity battles over defining images of self with their practitioners, they may also struggle against useful help and treatment that they might receive. They may remain autonomous but at costs to themselves as well as to relationships with their practitioners.

For some ill people, conflict with practitioners about the defining images of self has positive consequences. They not only become more attuned to their bodies, but become more self-conscious about how they wish to treat them. Through struggle and conflict, ill people who once acquiesced to negative self-definitions develop autonomous views of themselves and make autonomous decisions about their lives and their care. Although their motivation derived from proving the doctors wrong, they come to gain a sense of belief in themselves.

The problems inherent in the medical care system become apparent as illness worsens and as ill people are forced increasingly to rely upon it. This is the crucial turning point for ill people who have struggled valiantly for years to maintain control over their lives and to remain physically and financially independent. The fewer resources they have in money, help, and advocacy, the less likely they will be able to maintain some semblance of autonomy within the system. While self-advocacy may stave off the encroachments of the system upon autonomy for a time, it has obvious limits. Advocacy within the system, notably by nurses and social workers, helps. However, the narrowness of the system and the spiraling social, psychological, and economic needs of very sick people undermine the best efforts of concerned professionals to protect these patients' autonomy and to get them good care.[2]

The more dependent ill people become upon the health care system, the more likely losses of self accrue. For these people at this point, the medical care system takes on static, monolithic qualities. They depend upon the system for care—perhaps even for their very survival—but the system only provides care in narrow, rigid categories. Autonomy and independence dissolve at this point.

People with chronic illnesses bring knotty medical and social problems to their medical care professionals. The complex medical problems alone may defy a satisfactory solution. Many of the solutions to patients' problems lie beyond the medical care system—financial needs for housing, nutritious food, transportation, and prescriptions, social needs for assistance, fellowship, and purpose. Given the complexity of the patients' problems and the limited ability of the medical care system to deal with them, practitioners' frustration can be transposed to their patients. Hence, victim-blaming is a logical consequence of the current system of care.

What changes can be made in the system that would promote autonomy and, therefore, reduce loss of self? My argument takes the form of other critics of medical care but with a different twist on health (Conrad and Kern 1986; Crawford 1986; Zola 1986a). Perhaps most fundamental is the nature of the system itself; it is an illness care system founded in profits. What chronically ill people need is a *health* care system based upon *services*—diverse services. They need to preserve and to enhance their current health status. The system reinforces sickness over measures to maintain health *during* chronic illness. Insurance plans, the Medicare program, and often local hospital policies limit access and medical intervention until the chronically ill person's health has deteriorated into a crisis. Thus, the need for a system that protects health and prevents illness is perhaps even more pressing for chronically ill people than for the general public. The system does not provide a way for chronically ill people to regain, preserve, and maintain their health in comprehensive ways—even after they have suffered serious episodes. Granted, an isolated hospital might offer a cardiac or physical rehabilitation program. Similarly, a self-help group may plan excellent programs in a specific city. But elsewhere there may be no direct access to either rehabilitation or self-help.

Measures such as rehabilitation or patient education, when available at all, are usually available only for a brief period after a crisis. This poses severe limits for chronically ill people. Because learning about chronicity takes time and occurs during the tiny tasks and major hurdles of living their lives, ill people will often need information and help *after* they have left the medical setting. Furthermore, if practitioners give help or treatment when patients are ready for it, then they will be more likely to use it. They need to be able to enter and reenter the system repeatedly—and on their terms, not those of their practitioners.

Similarly, in keeping with a model of acute care, the system justifies continuing rehabilitation services on the basis of the patient's progress. Many chronically ill people will reach a level of functioning, for example in physical therapy, beyond which they do not improve. The system requires the patient's steady improvement. But chronically ill people must work just to stay where they are. Without the treatment and the social rewards of participating in it, they deteriorate—sometimes rapidly. Thus, chronically ill people need a system that furthers, rather than limits, their access to services.

Who needs the services? As it stands, the medical care system focuses on the individual who currently evinces the signs of sickness. By taking the ill individual as the unit of analysis, and therefore of service, the system ignores the social context of that individual. Hence, it also ignores the consequences of illness for other people within the person's social circle. An obvious consequence is the creation or acceleration of illness in overburdened caregivers. Less obvious are the conflict, emotional isolation, and resentment that can spread throughout families and destroy friendships. The system focuses on giving specialized care to one patient, or perhaps more accurately, to one part of the patient. Simultaneously, the problems accruing from serious chronic illness spread out through the patient's life and permeate his or her social world.

Thus, changing the system to support autonomy and to reduce losses of chronically ill people means producing a more open system with wider access, more comprehensive social, medical, and health services, and less medical dominance and fragmentation. These changes would help chronically ill people preserve their physical health, their relationships, their morale, and their autonomy. Subsequently, such changes would benefit the health of everyone.

Epilogue

What has happened to the people whose lives figured so promi-
nently at the beginning of each chapter? Where are they now?
As the book goes to press, the following stories about my respondents (appearing in the same order as in their respective
chapters) describe their lives at present.

Nancy Swenson continues to care for her mother who usually does not recognize her. But Nancy says that the care has
taken a toll on her health. Lately, she has developed a bad back,
a peptic ulcer, and diverticulitis. Recently, she had an emergency hospitalization for a mysterious and severe gastrointesti-
nal infection for which she is receiving more tests and from
which she has not recovered. Nancy says, "It's kind of scary
because God, what if it's a [cancerous] mass; is this the
carcinoid; is this *it?* . . . You think you're prepared, but you're
not." Nancy's doctor and new love both encourage her to relinquish her mother's care, so she has placed her name on a waiting list of a facility in another county that has a special unit for
Alzheimer's patients. Nancy hopes for a future as she and her
partner plan to move to a more rural area within commuting
distance of this facility. Despite all her added health problems,
Nancy finds more value and peace in her life now than ever
before.

Gloria Krause died three years ago after her bone marrow
replacement surgery. The surgery was actually successful, but
Gloria's body was drained. After the surgery, she never left the
intensive care ward. Her relationship with Greg had ended
three years before she died. During her last days, she asked
herself and her family, "Why did I give so much of my life to
Greg?" At her memorial service, a beautiful picture of Gloria

portrayed her with all the joy, spark, and radiance of the photographer's model she had always aspired to be.

Over the past three years, John Garston has become increasingly more reclusive. His closest companion, a feisty tomcat, was killed on the highway a few weeks ago and John feels the loss keenly. Except when a friend takes him to the grocery store, he does not leave the tiny cabin where he lives and works. With his discomfort, he no longer enjoys going to parties or even to antique auctions despite available rides. John managed to stop smoking, but his limited activity has steadily increased his weight. He knows that his condition has progressed and he acknowledges that a winter cold could kill him. Although he has frightening sporadic chest pains and increased belabored breathing, John still adamantly refuses to seek care or to be evaluated for SSI.

Harriet Binetti continues to live in her apartment with Sally. Harriet spends most of her days in bed now because she suffers from severe spasms due to the progression of her multiple sclerosis. However, she handles her confinement and discomfort stoically, and says, "It goes with the territory; it is just part of this disease." Harriet has much sorrow over her son's fate, for Robert is now dying with AIDS. She and Sally try to give him whatever help and support they can. Recently, he came to see them, and during the visit Sally took care of both Harriet and Robert.

After her long years of questioning the risks of intimacy, Sara Shaw has a happy marriage from which she is learning and growing. After the wedding, she moved to another state where her husband works. Their growing assortment of animals and the beauty of nature surround her on the small farm where they live. Sara expects her first child soon. Apparently, her pregnancy triggered a full-blown episode of mixed connective tissue disease, her first in years. Afterwards, her pregnancy proceeded well but, as she wrote, having the relapse was: "A reminder that I have a *chronic* disease."

Ann Rorty qualified for SSI, although she will be periodically reevaluated. Recently, she spent weeks in the hospital for a virus and is just beginning to recover from that. She says that she came close to death during that last hospitalization.

For two years, she has been involved with caring for her partner's parents, for whom she has much affection. His mother's Alzheimer's disease led to a recent institutionalization and his father's cancer has become terminal. Ann gave respite care so his father could do errands, cleaned their house, and spent time with both parents. Ann sees her future as uncertain because she has been so ill and because her partner looks forward to early retirement and traveling, a pursuit she feels that she could not share. She says that her heart disease has receded into the past since her current illness and continuing bowel problems are so much more pressing.

Tina Reidel still lives with the same man but perhaps with greater ease and comfort. Even though she struggles with arthritis daily, she continues to work and takes pride in her abilities. Tina changed jobs several years ago. Her current position requires her to impart accurate interpretations of insurance laws to people who usually are in crisis. She handles her work well and this supervisor values her. Pursuing her spiritual path has given Tina's life meaning and form. She makes the arduous trip to India to stay at the ashram when she can manage it financially and physically. Between participating in her spiritual group and receiving treatments from alternative healers, Tina seeks answers as to why she has arthritis and what she can do about it. She says, "Our own selves are the cause of all this stuff," and asks her chiropractor, "Why do you think I have so much pain?" Tina currently sees an acupuncturist, homeopathic practitioner, chiropractor, and a rheumatologist.

Mike Reilly continues to work as a salesman, a position he has held for a couple of years. The job means long hours on the road and a demanding daily schedule. Mike takes pride in representing the company's product and has appreciated having the job, especially since his employers had initial misgivings about hiring him due to his medical history. Mike works on commission so the vicissitudes of the larger economy can directly affect him. His daughters will soon be independent adults, which may ease things for him and his wife. Meanwhile, everyone in the family continues to have packed schedules and Mike continues his regular exercise program of walking.

During the last five years of his life, Mark Reinertsen found the loving friends he had longed for earlier. His best friends, a woman about his age and a young couple, remained steadfast in their care as his condition worsened. They provided emotional support, household help, and emergency transportation. Nonetheless, he died alone. During his last emergency hospitalization, Mark mistakenly gave his physician his friend's work number, rather than home number, but his crisis occurred on a weekend. Despite his physician's valiant attempts to locate her and hers to find Mark, he died before the mistake was remedied. Yet she felt that Mark may have intended to meet death alone as if completing a symbolic circle with his mother, for she, too, died alone with the same disease twenty-six years before. With Mark's death, his family history also died because he had been the lone survivor of his clan. Much more than being a dialysis patient, Mark's friends remember him for his humor, for his concern for humanity, and for his devotion to the peace movement. Mark would have wanted it that way.

Methodological Appendix

I began this study with the objective of furthering my knowledge about relationships between having a chronic illness, the self-concept, and experiencing time. From the beginning of this study, I planned to gather more data to illuminate, elaborate, and refine ideas that I had developed earlier in my dissertation (Charmaz 1973). My dissertation research had consisted of 55 qualitative interviews with 35 people. To obtain more data, I completed 115 additional intensive interviews with a new sample of 55 people with chronic illnesses. My data for this study primarily derive from these 115 formal interviews, although I have included several interview statements from my doctoral research. To buttress this data, I gathered a variety of research materials, including unpublished and published personal accounts, anecdotes, and observations. I also draw upon conversations and 20 informal interviews with caregivers and providers.

Because my earlier research had relied on referrals from physicians, who selected respondents they thought I ought to see, and because some of the interviews were conducted in hospitals, I sought referrals from other sources and talked with people in ordinary settings. To ensure that I would include people who avoided the medical care system, I sought referrals from colleagues, students, friends, and respondents as well as from professionals and illness support groups (Biernacki and Waldorf 1981).

My objectives led me first to seek interviewees who had a variety of serious chronic illnesses. The referral method allowed the participants to ask questions that they might have hesitated to ask me or to refuse to participate; however, only one person, who had a major setback just before the appointment, did so.

Ten individuals who learned of my work volunteered to participate. For example, a typist whom I found through a student
employment ad said that she had lupus erythematosus and offered to talk with me.

My criteria for the selecting interview participants included:
1) a diagnosis of a serious chronic but not terminal illness, 2) a
disease category that poses uncertainty, 3) present or past effects of the condition on the person's daily life, and 4) adult age
(twenty-one or older). The research criteria allowed for distinctions that individual participants did not always make, such as
including people who did not identify themselves as having a
chronic illness, or excluding individuals who had conditions
like minor arthritis, which did not substantially affect daily life.
I included illnesses like Hodgkin's lymphoma and breast cancer
since their survival rates have greatly lengthened. The major
disease categories in this study include cancer, circulatory diseases, colitis, renal failure, diabetes and metabolic diseases,
neurological conditions (multiple sclerosis, myasthenia gravis),
emphysema, and the collagen diseases (rheumatoid arthritis,
lupus erythematosus, idiopathic pulmonary fibrosis, mixed connective tissue disease, and Sjögren's syndrome).

The following demographic characteristics describe the 55
respondents at the time I first met them. Thirty-seven of the
interview respondents were women; 18 were men. I determined
social class status by the respondent's or their spouse's occupation and educational level. Accordingly, their social class levels
divided in the following categories: 9 upper middle class; 17
middle class; 7 working class, and 22 lower economic class
(including public or disability assistance). As could be expected when studying people with chronic illness longitudi-
nally, marked shifts in income occurred for some people over the
course of the research, and for others before the study. For example, two people who had been poor received sizable in-
heritances, which enabled them to adopt affluent middle-class
lifestyles. Several women who had been on welfare rejoined the
middle class through marriage. A few others, who had attended
college, graduated and got jobs. With but one exception, all of
the old women who were poor in late life had had working-or
middle-class lives. Several men retired early with a low income.

Sixteen individuals were between twenty-one and forty years of age; 24 were between forty and sixty; 7 were between sixty, and seventy, and 8 were over seventy. All the respondents were white. Twenty-six individuals had more than two years of college, 7 held advanced degrees, and 14 had finished high school; 8 had not. Twenty-eight people had partners or spouses. Eight people lived with children or roommates. Nine women and 3 men lived alone. Seven people resided in board and care institutions. Most interviews were conducted in the respondents' homes, although some took place at a dialysis unit, my office or home. All but one person agreed to be tape-recorded.

In this type of study, the researcher's methods of collecting data evolve while he or she is engaged in doing it. Because I already had collected a substantial amount of data and had a set of categories, my data collection methods for this study turned on obtaining materials that would shed further light on those categories. This approach to qualitative research, the grounded theory method, depends upon developing and refining the data collection tools *while* in the process of collecting the data (Charmaz 1983a; 1990; Glaser and Strauss 1967; Lofland and Lofland 1984; Strauss 1987). The grounded theory method and the elusive nature of my topics led me to seek multiple interviews from certain respondents. I chose people who faced uncertainty directly and were reflective about it. I wanted to follow people over months and years to see how, if at all, their views and experiences changed with the ebb and flow of their illnesses and of their lives.

Of the 55 respondents, I interviewed 26 people formally more than once. In turn, of those 26 respondents, I followed 16 men and women from five years to over a decade. I would have followed more had death or a move not intervened. Women were particularly hard to follow as they changed names, moved, or left the area entirely. Following people over time helps the researcher to see, discuss, and interpret the changes people define as their conditions improve, worsen, or stabilize. Further, multiple interviews also encourage a respondent to reveal private views of self, as he or she develops trust in the interviewer and comfort with the interviewing process.

Because I talked with a number of respondents multiple

times and sometimes saw them in a variety of other informal social settings, in certain respects the study edged toward participant observation. During this period, I attended several weddings as well as several memorial services of people I had interviewed. After we had talked four times, one person audited a university class I was teaching. A few respondents were friends or relatives of my friends and colleagues. I had tea with elderly women, visited elderly men, admired pictures of spouses, grandchildren, and boyfriends (in contrast, few of the male respondents were single), and met family members, friends, and housemates.

In keeping with the traditional logic of qualitative research, generally, and the grounded theory method, specifically, my research strategies differ from standard quantitative research design in two major ways. First, in the grounded theory method, the researcher uses his or her emerging analysis to direct the data collection. Hence, my interview questions developed in theoretical scope and usefulness during the course of the study. The questions reflected my deepening knowledge of the area, as well as growing skill as an interviewer. Second, the grounded theory methods place emphasis on developing theoretical analyses of the collected materials rather than on statistical verification procedures (Charmaz 1983a; 1990; Chenitz and Swanson 1986; Glaser 1978; Glaser and Strauss 1967; Strauss 1987; Strauss and Corbin 1990). Hence, I aimed to check and to refine my developing ideas by collecting specific data addressing those ideas. I designed an interview guide to explore both the respondent's experience and my ideas. Time and self are elusive topics to talk about; generally, illness is not. We only have a limited language with which to talk about time and self. To some extent, discussions about illness provide a vehicle for talking about time and self. In keeping with the difficulty of the topic, as well as with the analytic strategies of the grounded theory method, my questions evolved as I developed the analysis.

Given these topics, and my sense that not everyone can readily talk about them, I often could piece together beliefs and assumptions and taken-for-granted ways of acting. The more articulate or expressive men and women made more apparent what remained implicit with others. And people vary in how much they can talk about illness or about themselves, much less about meanings of time. One woman said that she had never talked so much about her illness to anyone. One man said that he had seldom talked so extensively or so deeply about himself. His statement and feelings provided me with a vivid reminder of how relative disclosures and explorations of feelings are. A moment before, I had thought to myself that he had skirted views and feelings, although he had given detailed information.

As a researcher, I sought to have people tell me about their lives from their perspectives rather than to force my preconceived interests and categories upon them. So I listened. I also believe that a researcher should not push the participant into an emotional abyss to grab interesting data and then leave. Thus, both the abstract level of the research topics and the potential emotional pain around illness necessitated being sensitive to how the topics and questions could affect a person. Once in a while, the interviews elicited tears and sadness. Many people remarked that the interview spurred them to reflect upon their lives or was therapeutic. Several people commented that they found me easy and safe to tell their feelings to. I told people to call me if they wanted to talk further, and occasionally a few of them did.

Usually, their stories tumbled out. Not uncommonly, one major question (such as "How are you now?") would elicit a fifteen-to-thirty-minute response. Later in the interview or in another interview, I asked specific questions. In keeping with the grounded theory method, these questions took into account areas and categories that I was developing. I discovered that participants could respond to abstract questions about self and time *if* they had thought about the issues posed by the question.

Some of the ideas discussed in the book are hard to explore through typical interview methods. But they can be pieced together from informal conversations, personal accounts, or witnessed during participant observation. For example, additional material about locating the self in the past can be gained from participant observation, for this process largely occurs without people's immediate awareness.

Although the grounded theory methods have been cast as

realist ethnography (Van Maanen 1988), what the method is seems to be taken as equivalent with how it has been used in earlier works (esp. Glaser and Strauss 1965;1967). It isn't equivalent. In this study, my use of grounded theory methods has a social constructionist, phenomenological, subjectivist cast because I emphasize lived experience throughout, offer "thick description" (Geertz 1973) of it, provide an interpretative rendering, and recognize that any such rendering comes from a particular point of view. As Clifford (1986; 1988), Marcus and Fischer (1986), and Richardson (1990) emphasize, the linguistic style of a work reflects the choices and assumptions of an author, which in turn reflect his or her training, interests, research decisions, relationship with the observed, and the historical and social context in which the study is completed.

Since I have detailed my analytic procedures elsewhere (Charmaz 1983a; 1990), I shall only outline them here. I began by exploring general research questions rather than by deducing a set of logically related hypotheses from a preexisting body of theory. As I gathered the data, I coded them for the respondent's assumptions, meanings, feelings, and actions. Instead of lumping responses into static topics, I tried to look for active processes and to discover how specific events and general processes were related. The coding process leads to making categories and analytically exploring them. By collecting more data on my developing categories, I expanded upon them and refined them. Throughout the study, I compared individuals' responses at different points in time, individuals with each other, and category to category. Throughout the analysis, I wrote memos to define and examine implicit ideas and processes that I saw in the data. These memos helped me to synthesize data and to define patterns within it. As the research ensued, my memos became more conceptual and abstract.

The grounded theory approach fosters following new leads and issues. For example, I had not realized the significance of disclosing illness until a number of people talked spontaneously of the problems they had with it. Then I went back and studied earlier interviews and formed new questions around it to ask others. The grounded theory approach aims to provide a dense set of social scientific concepts that define and explore processes. We assume that any portrayal of a process may change and should not be construed as final or as ultimate truth. In that spirit, I invite further exploration and refinement of the preceding analysis.

Notes

Chapter 1: Introduction

1. Rather than medicine as a social institution taking control of people's lives, medical practitioners become agents of much wider and interlocking institutions that have a powerful grasp over individual lives. Restrictive Medicaid regulations do not simply limit actions and choices of patients, and for that matter, practitioners; instead, they are coercive and punitive particularly toward patients. In this sense, the medicalization of life argument, though an important one, needs to take into account how economic and political constraints become imbedded in medical care and are played out in patients' lives. For illuminating discussions of the medicalization of life thesis, see Conrad and Schneider 1980; Zola 1986a.
2. Throughout the book, I use the terms "self" and "self-concept" interchangeably. A self-concept means the relatively stable, coherent *organization* of characteristics, attributes, attitudes, and sentiments that a person holds about himself or herself (Gecas 1982; Turner 1976). Because self-concepts consist of organized beliefs and feelings, they tend to change slowly. Self-images, in contrast, are fleeting images given in experience. But even these images are reflected through the mirror of interpretation of others' views of oneself. Not all self-images become part of the self-concept. But usually, repeated or crucial self-images eventually influence the self-concept.
3. Carlos Castenada's (1971) depiction of a separate reality of the magical culture of the Yaqui hearkens back to Schutz's (1971) conception of multiple realities. Denzin (1986) also observes that the world of the alcoholic is a separate reality.
4. For an examination of a journey with purpose and resolve, see Biernacki 1986. Biernacki traces the recovery from heroin addiction through addicts' resolve to make identity changes. His framework provides insight into the *processes* of identity change and the place of personal resolve in making them.
5. Thus the analysis that follows falls in the categories of reconstitution of self

with an emphasis on living with chronic illness (see Conrad 1987). In keeping with Conrad, I aim to make sociological conceptions of the illness experience. In contradistinction to Conrad's proposal (1987), I use different illnesses and the extent of them as the backdrop for comparisons between my *conceptual categories*, as analytically indicated, rather than making meaningful and explicit comparisons among illnesses on sociological grounds, as Conrad proposes. Surely, his proposal has value; it simply means a somewhat different research agenda and analytic venture than what I provide here.

6. Social scientific work, like other science, consists of stories, despite its positivistic trappings (Davis 1974). Any research is a product of the interactive processes between the observer and the observed and for that matter, between the observer and his or her discipline. Stripped of traditional disguise, the research process deals with creating the data, compiling it, and conferring meaning upon it.

7. A caveat. To portray the feeling of experiences and events, I sometimes write as if those experiences and events had monolithic properties. They do not. Similarly, I may seem to argue that time acts—such as moving, slowing, or stopping. It does not. But people's perceptions of change and meaning are expressed in their views of time. Part of those perceptions are the feelings that emerge in these people's experience of time while they are ill. The melding of feeling and time into *a* reality, rather than *the* reality is what I wish to portray.

Chapter 2: Chronic Illness as Interruption

1. For a more complete discussion of the sick role, see Gerhardt 1989; Gordon 1966; Segall 1976; Siegler and Osmond 1979; and Twaddle 1969. The acute illness and care model inherent in the concept of the sick role is shared by many practitioners as well as patients.

2. Turner (1976) observes that people do not adopt all of their attributes and characteristics into their self-concepts. Rather, they are selective. It follows that ill people, particularly in the early stages of illness, will base their concepts of their "real" selves on other attributes than illness.

3. Of course, someone else might so resent lack of acknowledgment from a spouse that none of the positive consequences above could have been realized.

Chapter 3: Intrusive Illness

1. My argument takes ill people's definitions as the point of departure. I do not negate the existence of disease processes. I do take note of how people recognize and act upon those disease processes and treat them as "illness."

2. This woman's views of illness come close to Herzlich's (1973) concept of illness as a destroyer, with the subsequent logic of distinguishing between remaining active and not being ill, merging self and activity, and valuing self in activity. See R.G.A. Williams's (1981 a and b) explication of logical analysis. At the time of her comment, Vera Mueller was a Medi-Cal patient. She talked about her extreme reluctance to make use of the service because she could not stand the possibility of being seen as abusing the welfare system. Conceivably then, her views of and experiences within the Medi-Cal system contribute to her definition of illness.

3. Though some people show concern for disease control, most place greater emphasis on the consequences of symptoms for their ability to function today and tomorrow rather than in consideration for years or decades into the future (see also Strauss et al. 1984).

4. Acceptance of illness is often taken by practitioners as a prerequisite for being able to move beyond it. We need to look at who makes the assessment of acceptance. Whose terms are accepted? Why? Acceptance is also couched in evaluations of compliance to practitioners' programs and advice (see also Charmaz 1980b).

5. By doing so, ill people may reduce the intensity of bad days and keep them more distant from self.

6. The differences in attitudes between very old and younger individuals may represent social class, rather than age differences. Most very old people belong to the working class because education and opportunity were the purview of the privileged when they were young. Many of the very old were immigrants or the sons and daughters of immigrants. In 1980, less than half of those over eighty-five had completed one year of high school; almost one-third did not complete eighth grade (see Bould, Sanborn, and Reif 1989).

Chapter 4: Immersion in Illness

1. A blurring of spatial arrangements may blur progressive immersion in illness. Without the customary markers of days and hours in a conventional workplace, for example, ill people may not realize how their lives have changed.

2. In this sense, illness reveals uncertainty and instability in a world previously taken for granted as predictable and stable. Illness also undermines or destroys beliefs in the ability of the individual to *control* threats to the self (Kidel 1988).

3. The smoothness of a repeated regimen itself can become a marker of the self and a sign that nothing worse is happening with the illness. Not uncommonly, therefore, people take refuge in their regimens; they are a safe place to situate the self. The regimen takes on its own rhythm, a cyclical rather than a linear rhythm (cf. Young 1988). Of course, the efficacy of the regimen may remain untested.

4. Sourkes (1982) calls it "neutral time," perhaps to indicate the lack of move-ment; however, though bland for some people, this uncertain, ambiguous experience of time is not bland for others. Further, though illness may seem quiescent during this period, the ill person may become aware of the slightest nuances of change.

5. The mechanical repetition of the same day is at odds with the rapid se-quencing of events that we associate with youth. For young people who tied self-worth to activity and diversity, being ill primarily meant a series of losses. In addition, creating meaning while experiencing unchanging time taxes anyone who holds a linear progressive view of time.

6. Some ill people had been at the centers of their family and friendship circles; they had focused on others and their needs for years. They may infuriate their family and friends when they no longer do so. Then they are likely to become depressed, apathetic, and withdrawn—quietly pas-sive. Sometimes relatives will attempt to intervene with an elder's turning inward to self when they view doing so as taking permanent leave of them.

Chapter 5: Disclosing Illness

1. Throughout the chapter, I focus on disclosing, although I note where disclosing fits with other forms of telling and how it compares with them.

2. Certainly, all the ways of telling make more or less use of impression management. Hence, people move from controlling highly manipulative and strategic performances to making mental plans about how to inform effectively. See Schlenker 1980 for a discussion of varied uses of impres-sion management.

3. Hochschild (1983) discusses the commercialization of feeling with man-aged emotions that benefit the corporate owners, rather than the workers. The logical extension of her argument might lead one to advocate express-ing feelings. However, ill people often find that expressing anger leads to more anger; expressing self-pity generates more self-pity, etc. (cf. Tavris 1982). Even if ill people internalize feeling rules that call for limiting emo-tional expression, they still may say that they "feel better" about not letting their feelings show.

Chapter 6: Living with Chronic Illness

1. The health care system separates people from each other, encourages them to see illness as a private problem, and fosters independent and individual-ized, rather than shared, learning about the disease and how to live with it. Irving K. Zola (1986b) makes a similar point in his review of Locker's *Disabil-*

ity and Disadvantage. He states à la Parsons (1953) that a function of the doctor-patient relationship is to contain the spread of deviance; therefore, patients are kept isolated from each other. As Zola points out, the Independent Living Movement has made substantial inroads in reducing isolation, sharing information, and eliminating barriers to full participation. The other notable movement in which patients take control of their care and shared medical knowledge is, of course, the women's health movement. See Ruzek (1979) for the history of that movement. In contrast, I argue that the hospice movement differs since it has moved to become more thoroughly imbedded in the established medical care system (Charmaz 1980b).

2. I am indebted to Barbara Rosenblum for clarifying this point.
3. Pinder (1988) also has observed the process of making trade-offs to accomplish goals and tasks among people with Parkinson's disease. She points out that the trade-offs they make are without a stable foundation. An uncertain course of illness can vitiate efforts to create a balanced life, despite whatever trade-offs are made.
4. Attending a community dining site for the elderly may prompt older people to regain community standards of cleanliness, which they had lost for months or years. Their peers may prod unkempt elders to attend to themselves with questions like: "What's that spot on your blouse?"
5. Irving K. Zola made a similar point in his presentation, "Aging and Disability," given at Sonoma State University, February 3, 1987.
6. Corbin and Strauss (1988) also found the domino effect in their study of chronically ill and disabled people.

Chapter 7: Time Perspectives and Time Structures

1. Ill people's time perspectives shift according to the meanings that they attach to their illness, the way that they experience it, their "life structure" (Levinson et al. 1978), their age, and whether or not they can merge the illness into their daily routine. Idler (1979) states that "Sickness creates and measures its own time." Yes, under certain conditions, it does. These conditions include: 1) acknowledging sickness, 2) contrasting present sickness and past perceived wellness, or quiescence, and 3) observing when life becomes structured around illness. Otherwise, sickness does not create and measure its own time at all unless and until the person feels overcome and swept away by it.
2. Living one day at a time takes work. Doing so especially takes work when, otherwise, fear and loss would overwhelm the person. See Lewis (1985).
3. Certainly living one day at a time is not limited to ill people. The strategy has long been used by recovering alcoholics. Healthy people also adopt the strategy when feeling overwhelmed by their situations.
4. I am indebted to Anna Hazan for this anecdote. Personal communication, September 23, 1988.

Chapter 8: Timemarkers and Turning Points

1. This stance comes close to what Maines and Hardesty (1987) call a linear temporal world. Here, people are concerned with what they need to do and pay less attention to or disregard the possibility that their futures are now contingent.

2. Anniversaries are long remembered and may be honored. Cousins (1983) tells of a woman who visited him who wanted to start a support organization for cancer patients. She had had an episode of cancer ten years before. After her tenth anniversary of the initial report, she declared herself free of cancer. Anniversaries also may linger in mood though the marker itself is forgotten. Hall (1983) reports that each spring he suffers from a lingering depression. Years later he realized that his depression emanated from the collapse of his parents' marriage and the departure of his mother from the family.

3. Couch (1982) makes a similar point when he observes that the past can be forgotten, selectively remembered, or reconstructed.

4. Lewis (1971) argues that shame is an emotion that is blamed on another. Not necessarily. Another person may evoke feelings of shame, under certain conditions. But when feelings are ambiguous and the boundaries of the self are open, then shame may become an overriding emotion. Knowledge of community standards alone, without the actual presence of another individual, can give rise to shame. For an explication of shame as a master emotion, see Scheff 1989; 1990.

Chapter 9: The Self in Time

1. This loss is often implicit, though understood by ill people who believe that they have left the world of active, productive adults. Nursing home patients particularly may lose their connecting links to people outside the institution, as they become a part of the institutional reality.

2. Mishler (1986) offers a comprehensive discussion of the construction of narratives and of their reconstruction by social scientists.

3. For discussions of the meaning of duration, see also Flaherty 1987, Mead 1934, and Sharron 1982.

4. Lopata (1986) provides the insight that a life review not only stretches back into the past, but also may stretch into the future.

Chapter 10: Lessons from the Experience of Illness

1. I overstate the distinction here between reason as the basis of autonomy and emotion as underlying control for purposes of contrast. Clearly,

demonstrating autonomy is not stripped of feeling, nor does maintaining control occur without reasoning. They simply represent more or less feeling and reasoning. Presumably, as people gain autonomy, their actions reflect conscious reasoning.

2. It is important to distinguish between advocacy and intervention here. Many professional interventions do not reflect advocacy. Despite being well intended *for* the patient, the actions do not derive *from* the patients' goals and priorities. Rather, these actions derive from the professional's sense of what can, and often should, be done.

Glossary

Apnea. A temporary state of not breathing; it often occurs during sleep among adults (sleep apnea).

Board and Care. Residential care; a level of institutional care providing residents with a room (often shared), meals, and some supervision of nonmedical personal care. These facilities usually do not offer nursing services. They may not have twenty-four-hour supervision, although many do. Frail elderly and younger people with disabilities live in these facilities, which are private or paid through Social Security supplemental income.

Carcinoid Syndrome. A complex of symptoms, including flushing of the skin, diarrhea, abdominal cramps, valvular heart disease, and cyanosis, which are caused by vasoactive secretions of metastatic small tumors usually in the intestinal area. These tumors are extremely difficult to locate during surgery. Survival rates after diagnosis range from two to twenty years.

Cerebral Vascular Accident (CVA). A general term to indicate abrupt blockage with resulting insufficient cerebral circulation or hemorrhage in the brain. In either case, the resulting neurological deficits reflect the area of the brain that is damaged. The ischemic lesions are commonly referred to as strokes. Common residuals include paralysis, weakness, or loss of sensation on one side of the body, loss of speech and language skills, impaired reasoning, facial paralysis, emotional lability, personality changes, and depression.

Chronic Fatigue Syndrome. A cluster of symptoms including debilitating fatigue that remains unrelieved by bed rest, reduces the individual's daily activity by 50 percent, and

287

cannot be attributed to any other condition (Fisher et al. 1989).

Colitis. An episodic or chronic inflamation of the colon characterized by abdominal pain, constipation, and diarrhea. Some people do not experience pain but have sudden, urgent, uncontrollable episodes of diarrhea during or immediately following a meal.

Diabetes. A common chronic metabolic disorder resulting from insufficient production or function of insulin. Symptoms include weight loss, excessive thirst and urination, and the presence of sugar in the blood and urine. Type I diabetes usually has an onset in youth and results in requiring injections of insulin. Type II is adult-onset and may be precipitated by obesity, pregnancy, and stress as well as heredity. Mild forms may be handled by diet, rest, and exercise. In both types, serious complications can cause atherosclerosis, coronary artery disease, ulcers and gangrene of the feet, blindness, kidney failure, and peripheral neuropathies.

Discoid Lupus. A chronic disorder, probably autoimmune in origin, primarily affecting the skin with characteristic butterfly-shaped lesions across the cheeks and bridge of the nose. Patients are often photosensitive.

Emphysema. An abnormal condition of the lungs in which the air spaces of the lung enlarge, accompanied by destructive changes of the walls of the alveoli resulting in decreased respiratory function. Symptoms include shortness of breath, labored breathing, cough, rapid heart rate, with subsequent restlessness, weakness, and confusion as the disease progresses and the brain does not receive enough oxygen. Pulmonary edema and congestive heart failure are common complications.

Environmental Illness. A severe sensitivity to ordinary chemicals and pollutants that can trigger exhaustion, respiratory disorders, neurological symptoms such as disorientation, neuromuscular dysfunction, and disability, and life-threatening heart arrythmias. People with these symptoms often describe themselves as allergic to traffic fumes, natural gas, mildew, paints, carpets, synthetic fabrics, and plastics. They strip their homes of such materials and may seek housing in areas without pollution. Their illnesses are controversial and largely unrecognized by medical professionals. Many allergists believe that the illness is psychosomatic rather than allergic in origin.

Exacerbation. A flare-up of symptoms; an increase in the progression of a disease.

General Assistance (Public Assistance). Extremely limited welfare assistance for impoverished adults.

Hodgkin's Lymphoma. A malignant disease of unknown cause characterized by cellular changes and enlargement of lymph node tissue. It may occur in localized areas or throughout the body, and it may vary in rate of progression. The symptoms include enlarged lymph nodes, fatigue, generalized itching, low-grade fever, loss of weight, night sweats, and pain when there is bone involvement. Radiation and/or chemotherapy produce lengthy remissions in many cases and long survival rates in most cases with limited disease.

Iatrogenic Effect. A condition caused by diagnostic procedures, medical treatments, and medical or surgical interventions or by contact with medical settings or staff.

Idiopathic Pulmonary Fibrosis. A disease of unknown origin in which there is a substantial increase of fibrous connective tissue in the lungs. It leads to fatigue, weakness, shortness of breath, and labored breathing.

Illness Trajectory. The temporal course of the disease and the work and relationships involved in controlling or shaping this course (Corbin and Strauss 1988).

Lupus Erythematosus (Systemic Lupus Erythematosus). An inflammatory connective tissue disease that affects the vital organs as well as the joints and central nervous system. Lupus patients experience high fatigue, arthritis and arthralgia, cutaneous lesions, and, often, photosensitivity. They frequently have recurrent pleurisy, enlarged lymph glands, inflammation of the pericardium, central nervous system involvement, and progressive renal failure.

Medicaid Program. The federally supported and state administered medical assistance program for those in need. Uninsured individuals, primarily low-income elders and those eligible for other public programs, who meet the stringent Medicaid eligibility requirements, receive treatment through this program.

Medi-Cal Program. The California Medicaid program.

Medicare. The federally supported catastrophic medical care insurance program available to elderly people who are covered by Social Security. This program requires private, or if the individual is eligible, public copayment for services, which primarily cover acute episodes.

Mixed Connective Tissue Disease. A rheumatic disease of unknown etiology, thought to be autoimmune in nature, with overlapping characteristics of several connective tissue diseases such as Raynaud's phenomena, swollen hands with sausage-like fingers, weakness and wasting of muscles close to the body, fever, rashes, joint pain and swelling, esophageal abnormalities, pulmonary involvement, and cardiac symptoms. Some patients have lengthy remissions although proliferative vascular lesions can lead to death.

Multiple Sclerosis. An autoimmune disease in which the nerves of the central nervous system lose their myelin sheath in patches, which results in multiple neurological symptoms such as loss of balance, double vision, partial blindness, pain in the eye, emotional lability, lack of judgment, forgetfulness, tremors, spasticity, numbness, paralysis, incontinence, and fatigue. It is an unpredictable disease characterized by remissions and exacerbations that eventually lead to permanent disability.

Myasthenia Gravis. An autoimmune disease characterized by muscular weakness due to abnormal neuromuscular transmission. The course of the disease varies, ranging from mild involvement to life-threatening respiratory crisis.

Peripheral Neuropathy. An abnormal condition affecting the nerves outside the central nervous system, which causes sensory, motor, reflex, and vasomotor symptoms.

Photodermatitis. An unusual inflammation of the skin due to only brief exposure (minutes) to the sun. Photodermatitis is characteristic in people who have lupus erythematosus.

Premature Ventricular Contraction (PVC). An irregular cardiac rhythm that may not be medically significant when only an isolated occurrence but much more significant when frequent and recurrent. These PVC's typically indicate cardiac abnormality and sometimes precede ventricular fibrillation, which, in turn, leads to unconsciousness and possible sudden death unless life-saving interventions are administered.

Public Assistance. See General Assistance.

Raynaud's Phenomena. An abnormal condition in which the arteries and arterioles (usually of the fingers) spasm, producing a bluish color as oxygen is greatly reduced. It often occurs in conjunction with connective tissue disorders.

Remission. A quiescent phase during which the symptoms partially or completely fade.

Sjögren's Syndrome. A chronic, systemic, inflammatory disease of the mucuous membranes with characteristic drying of the eyes, nose, and mouth. Although it is of unknown origin, it is believed to be an autoimmune disease and often accompanies rheumatoid arthritis or lupus erythematosus. Taste and smell may be lost. Teeth may also be lost. The dryness of the respiratory system readily leads to infections and pneumonias. Chronic liver and pancreatic disease often follow. The incidence of lymphoma is greatly increased in people who have Sjögren's syndrome.

Supplemental Security Income (SSI). A federally supported and state assisted income transfer program for impoverished elderly and disabled people who cannot work and who meet extensive eligibility requirements.

References

Aaronson, Bernard S. 1972. "Behavior and the Place Names of Time." In *The Future of Time*, ed. Henri Yaker, Humphry Osmond, and Frances Cheek, 405–438. Garden City, N.Y.: Doubleday.

Albrecht, Gary L., and Judith A. Levy. 1984. "A Sociological Perspective of Physical Disability." In *Advances in Medical Social Science*, ed. Julio L. Ruffini, 45–105. New York: Gordon and Breach.

Alonzo, Angelo. 1979. "Everyday Illness Behavior: A Situational Approach to Health Status Deviations." *Social Science and Medicine* 13:397–404.

Anderson, Robert. 1988. "The Quality of Life of Stroke Patients and Their Careers." In *Living with Chronic Illness*, ed. Robert Anderson and Michael Bury, 14–42. London: Unwin Hyman.

Barber, Bernard. 1983. *The Logic and Limits of Trust*. New Brunswick, N.J.: Rutgers University Press.

Barley, Stephen R. 1988. "On Technology, Time and Social Order: Technologically Induced Change in the Temporal Organization of Radiological Work." In *Making Time: Ethnographies of High-Technology Organizations*, ed. Frank A. Dubinskas, 123–169. Philadelphia: Temple University Press.

Baszanger, Isabelle. 1989. "Pain: Its Experience and Treatments." *Social Science and Medicine* 29:425–434.

Becker, Ernest. 1975. "Socialization, Command of Performance and Mental Illness." In *Life As Theatre: A Dramaturgical Sourcebook*, ed. Dennis Brissett and Charles Edgley, 292–301. Chicago: Aldine.

Becker, Howard S. 1960. "Notes on the Concept of Commitment." *American Journal of Sociology* 66:32–40.

Becker, Howard S., Blanche Geer, Everett C. Hughes, and Anselm L. Strauss. 1961. *Boys in White: Student Culture in Medical School*. Chicago: University of Chicago Press.

Biernacki, Patrick. 1986. *Pathways from Heroin Addiction: Recovery without Treatment*. Philadelphia: Temple University Press.

Biernacki, Patrick, and Dan Waldorf. 1981. "Snowball Sampling: Problems and Techniques of Chain Referral Sampling." *Sociological Methods and Research* 10:141–163.

Birrer, Cynthia. 1979. *Multiple Sclerosis: A Personal View.* Springfield, Ill.: Charles C. Thomas.

Blumer, Herbert. 1969. *Symbolic Interactionism.* Englewood Cliffs, N.J.: Prentice-Hall.

Bould, Sally, Beverly Sanborn, and Laura Reif. 1989. *Eighty-five Plus: The Oldest Old.* Belmont, Calif.: Wadsworth.

Brody, Elaine. 1985. "Parent Care as a Normative Family Stress." *Gerontologist* 15:19–29.

Brody, Howard. 1987. *Stories of Sickness.* New Haven: Yale University Press.

Brooks, Nancy A., and Ronald R. Matson. 1982. "Social-Psychological Adjustment to Multiple Sclerosis." *Social Science and Medicine* 16:2129–2135.

———. 1987. "Managing Multiple Sclerosis." In *Research in the Sociology of Health Care: The Experience and Management of Chronic Illness,* ed. Julius A. Roth and Peter Conrad, 6:73–106. Greenwich, Conn.: JAI Press.

Bury, Michael. 1982. "Chronic Illness as Disruption." *Sociology of Health and Illness* 4:167–182.

———. 1988. "Meanings at Risk: The Experience of Arthritis." In *Living with Chronic Illness,* ed. Robert Anderson and Michael Bury, 89–116. London: Unwin Hyman.

Calkins, Kathy. 1970. "Time: Perspectives, Marking and Styles of Usage." *Social Problems* 17:487–501.

———. 1972. "Shouldering a Burden." *Omega* 3:16–32.

Calland, Chad H. 1972. "Iatrogenic Problems in End-Stage Renal Failure." *The New England Journal of Medicine* 287:334–336.

Calnan, Michael. 1987. *Health & Illness: The Lay Perspective.* London: Tavistock.

Cassell, Eric J. 1983. "What is the Function of Medicine?" In *Moral Problems in Medicine,* ed. Samuel Gorowitz, Ruth Macklin, Andrew L. Jameton, John M. O'Connor, and Susan Sherwin, 73–77. Englewood Cliffs, N.J.: Prentice-Hall.

Castenada, Carlos. 1971. *A Separate Reality.* New York: Simon & Schuster.

Charmaz, Kathy, 1973. "Time and Identity: The Shaping of Selves of the Chronically Ill." Ph.D. diss., University of California, San Francisco.

———. 1977. "Time and the Structure of the Self." Unpublished manuscript.

———. 1980a. "The Social Construction of Self-Pity in the Chronically Ill." In *Studies in Symbolic Interaction,* ed. Norman K. Denzin, 3:123–146. Greenwich, Conn.: JAI Press.

———. 1980b. *The Social Reality of Death.* Reading, Mass.: Addison-Wesley.

———. 1981. "Time and the Structure of the Self." Paper presented at the Pacific Sociological Association, Portland, March. 18–21.

———. 1983a. "The Grounded Theory Method: An Explication and Interpretation." In *Contemporary Field Research,* ed. Robert M. Emerson, 109–126. Boston: Little-Brown.

———. 1983b. "Loss of Self: A Fundamental Form of Suffering in the Chronically Ill." *Sociology of Health & Illness* 5:168–195.

———. 1984. "Intrusive Illness: Meanings and Experiences of Chronic Illness." Paper presented at the Pacific Sociological Association, Seattle, April 11–14.

———. 1985a. "Experiencing Chronic Illness as an Interruption." Paper presented at the Society for the Study of Symbolic Interaction, Washington, August 23–26.

———. 1985b. "Socializing Others to One's Illness." Paper presented at the Pacific Sociological Association, Albuquerque, April 17–20.

———. 1986. "The Emotional Implications of Chronic Illness for Women." Paper presented at the Eleventh World Congress of Sociology, New Delhi, August 18–23.

———. 1987. "Struggling for a Self: Identity Levels of the Chronically Ill." In *Research in the Sociology of Health Care: The Experience and Management of Chronic Illness*, ed. Julius A. Roth and Peter Conrad, 6:283–321. Greenwich, Conn.: JAI Press.

———. 1989. "The Self in Time." In *Studies in Symbolic Interaction*, ed. Norman K. Denzin, 10:127–141. Greenwich, Conn.: JAI Press.

———. 1990. "Discovering Chronic Illness: Using Grounded Theory." *Social Science and Medicine* 30:1161–1172.

Chenitz, W. Carol, and Janice M. Swanson. 1986. *From Practice to Grounded Theory: Qualitative Research in Nursing*. Reading, Mass.: Addison-Wesley.

Chester, Laura. 1987. *Lupus Novice: Toward Self Healing*. Barrytown, N.Y.: Station Hill Press.

Cioran, E. M. 1970. *The Fall Into Time*. Chicago: Quadrangle Books.

Clark, Matt, with Holly Morris, Patricia King, Pamela Abramson, Mariana Gosnell, Mary Hager, Barbara Burgower, and Janet Huck. 1985. "Living with Cancer." *Newsweek*. April 8:64–77.

Clark, Robert E., and Emily E. La Beff. 1982. "Death Telling: Managing the Delivery of Bad News." *Journal of Health and Social Behavior* 23:366–380.

Clarke, Adele. 1982. "The Ambiguous Condition: Patients' Experience of Cervical Dysplasia." Paper presented at the Society for the Study of Social Problems, San Francisco, August 3–5.

Clifford, James. 1986. "Introduction: Partial Truths." In *Writing Culture*, ed. James Clifford and George E. Marcus, 1–26. Berkeley, Calif.: University of California Press.

———. 1988. *The Predicament of Culture*. Cambridge: Harvard University Press.

Cobb, Ann Kuckelman, and Edna Hamera. 1986. "Illness Experience in a Chronic Disease—ALS." *Social Science and Medicine* 23:641–650.

Cogswell, Betty E. 1968. "Self-socialization: Readjustment of Paraplegics in the Community." *Journal of Rehabilitation* 34:11–13.

Comaroff, Jean, and Peter Maguire. 1981. "Ambiguity and the Search for Meaning: Childhood Leukemia in the Modern Clinical Context." *Social Science and Medicine* 15:115–123.

Conrad, Peter. 1985. "The Meaning of Medications: Another Look at Compliance." *Social Science and Medicine* 20:28–37.

———. 1987. "The Experience of Illness: Recent and New Directions." In *Research in the Sociology of Health Care: The Experience and Management of Chronic Illness*, ed. Julius A. Roth and Peter Conrad, 6:1–32. Greenwich, Conn.: JAI Press.

Conrad, Peter, and Rochelle Kern. 1986. "General Introduction." In *The Sociology of Health and Illness: Critical Perspectives*, ed. Peter Conrad and Rochelle Kern, 1–5. New York: St. Martin's.

Conrad, Peter, and Joseph W. Schneider. 1980. *Deviance and Medicalization: From Badness to Sickness*. St. Louis: Mosby.

Cooley, Charles H. 1902. *Human Nature and Social Order*. New York: Charles Scribner's Sons.

Corbin, Juliet M., and Anselm L. Strauss. 1984. "Collaboration: Couples Working Together to Manage Chronic Illness." *Image* 4:109–115.

———. 1985. "Managing Chronic Illness at Home: Three Lines of Work." *Qualitative Sociology* 8:224–247.

———. 1988. *Unending Work and Care: Managing Chronic Illness at Home*. San Francisco: Jossey-Bass.

Cornwell, Jocelyn. 1984. *Hard-earned Lives*. London: Tavistock.

Couch, Carl J. 1982. "Temporality and Paradigms of Thought." In *Studies in Symbolic Interaction*, ed. Norman K. Denzin, 4:1–24. Greenwich, Conn.: JAI Press.

———. 1989. *Social Processes and Relationships: A Formal Approach*. Dix Hills, N.Y.: General Hall.

Cousins, Norman. 1983. *The Healing Heart: Antidotes to Panic and Helplessness*. New York: Avon.

Cowie, Bill. 1976. "The Patient's Perception of His Heart Attack." *Social Science and Medicine* 10:87–96.

Cozby, Paul C. 1973. "Self-Disclosure: A Literature Review." *Psychological Bulletin* 79:73–91.

Crawford, Robert. 1986. "Individual Responsibility and Health Politics." In *The Sociology of Health and Illness: Critical Perspectives*, ed. Peter Conrad and Rochelle Kern, 369–377. New York: St. Martin's.

Dahlberg, Charles Clay, and Joseph Jaffe. 1977. *Stroke: A Doctor's Personal Story of His Recovery*. New York: Norton.

Davis, Fred. 1961. "Deviance Disavowal: The Management of Strained Interaction by the Visibly Handicapped." *Social Problems* 9:120–132.

———. 1963. *Passage Through Crisis: Polio Victims and Their Families*. Indianapolis: Bobbs-Merrill.

———. 1974. "Stories and Sociology." *Urban Life and Culture*. 3:310–316.

———. 1979. *Yearning for Yesterday: A Sociology of Nostalgia*. New York: Free Press.

Davis, Marcella. 1973. *Living with Multiple Sclerosis*. St. Louis: Charles C. Thomas.

De Grazia, Sebastian. 1962. *Of Time, Work, and Leisure*. New York: Twentieth Century Fund.

DeMille, Agnes. 1981. *Reprieve*. New York: Doubleday.

Denzin, Norman K. 1980. "A Phenomenology of Emotion and Deviance." *Zeilschrift für Soziologie* 9:251–261.

———. 1982. "On Time and Mind." In *Studies in Symbolic Interaction*, ed. Norman K. Denzin, 5:35–43. Greenwich, Conn.: JAI Press.

———. 1984. *On Understanding Emotion*. San Francisco: Jossey-Bass.

———. 1986. *The Alcoholic Self*. Beverly Hills, Calif.: Sage.

———. 1987. "Under the Influence of Time: Reading the Interactional Text." *Sociological Quarterly* 28:327–341.

———. 1989. *Interpretative Interactionism*. Newbury Park, Calif.: Sage.

Derlaga, Valerian J., and Janusz Grzelak. 1979. "Appropriateness of Self-Disclosure." In *Self-Disclosure*, ed. Gordon T. Chelune et al., 151–176. San Francisco: Jossey-Bass.

Dubinskas, Frank A. 1988. "Cultural Construction: The Many Faces of Time." In *Making Time: Ethnographies of High-Technology Organizations*, ed. Frank A. Dubinskas, 3–38. Philadelphia: Temple University Press.

Durkheim, Emile. 1951. *Suicide*. Glencoe, Ill.: Free Press.

Duval, M. Louise. 1984. "Psychosocial Metaphors of Physical Distress Among MS Patients." *Social Science and Medicine* 19:635–638.

Fabrega, Horacio Jr., and Peter K. Manning. 1972. "Disease, Illness, and Deviant Careers." In *Theoretical Perspectives on Deviance*, ed. Robert A. Scott and Jack D. Douglas, 93–116. New York: Basic Books.

Fagerhaugh, Shizuko. 1975. "Getting Around with Emphysema." In *Chronic Illness and the Quality of Life*, ed. Anselm L. Strauss and Barney G. Glaser, 99–107. St. Louis: Mosby.

Fagerhaugh, Shizuko, and Anselm L. Strauss. 1977. *Politics of Pain Management*. Reading, Mass.: Addison-Wesley.

Feil, Naomi. 1985. "Resolution: The Final Life Task." *Journal of Humanistic Psychology* 25:91–105.

Fiore, Niel A. 1984. *The Road Back to Health*. New York: Bantam.

Fisher, Gregg Charles, with Stephen E. Straus, Paul R. Cheney, and James M. Oleske, 1987. *Chronic Fatigue Syndrome*. New York: Warner Books.

Flaherty, Michael G. 1987. "Multiple Realities and the Experience of Duration." *Sociological Quarterly* 28:313–326.

Fraisse, Paul. 1984. "Perception and Estimation of Time." In *Annual Review of Psychology*, ed. M. R. Rosenzweig and L. W. Porter, 35:1–36. Palo Alto, Calif.: Annual Reviews.

Gadow, Sally. 1982. "Body and Self: A Dialectic." In *The Humanity of the Ill*, ed. Victor Kestenbaum, 86–100. Knoxville: University of Tennessee Press.

———. 1983. "Frailty and Strength: The Dialectic in Aging." *Gerontologist* 23:144–147.

Gecas, Viktor. 1982. "The Self-concept." *Annual Review of Sociology* 8:1–33.

Geertz, Clifford. 1973. *The Interpretation of Cultures*. New York: Basic Books.

———. 1988. *Works and Lives: The Anthropologist as Author*. Stanford, Calif.: Stanford University Press.

Gerhardt, Uta. 1979. "Coping and Social Action: Theoretical Reconstruction of the Life-event Approach." *Sociology of Health & Illness* 1:195–225.

———. 1989. *Ideas about Illness.* New York: New York University Press.

Gerhardt, Uta, and Marianne Brieskorn-Zinke. 1986. "The Normalization of Hemodialysis at Home." In *Research in the Sociology of Health Care: The Adoption and Social Consequences of Medical Technologies,* ed. Julius A. Roth and Sheryl B. Ruzek, 4:271–317. Greenwich, Conn.: JAI Press.

Gerson, Elihu. 1976. "The Quality of Life." *American Sociological Review* 41:793–806.

Glaser, Barney G. 1966. "Disclosure of Terminal Illness." *Journal of Health and Human Behavior* 7:83–91.

———. 1978. *Theoretical Sensitivity.* Mill Valley, Calif.: The Sociology Press.

Glaser, Barney G., and Anselm L. Strauss. 1965. *Awareness of Dying.* Chicago: Aldine.

———. 1967. *The Discovery of Grounded Theory.* Chicago: Aldine.

———. 1968. *Time for Dying.* Chicago: Aldine.

Goffman, Erving. 1959. *The Presentation of Self in Everyday Life.* Garden City, N.Y.: Doubleday.

———. 1961a. *Asylums.* Garden City, N.Y.: Doubleday.

———. 1961b. *Encounters.* New York: Bobbs-Merrill.

———. 1963. *Stigma.* Englewood Cliffs, N.J.: Prentice-Hall.

———. 1967. *Interaction Ritual.* New York: Pantheon.

———. 1975. *Strategic Interaction.* New York: Ballantine.

Gold, Steven J. 1983. "Getting Well: Impression Management as Stroke Rehabilitation." *Qualitative Sociology* 6:238–254.

Goodvage, Maria. 1988. "I Get So Lonely Out Here." *This World, San Francisco Chronicle.* November 27, 15.

Gordon, Gerald. 1966. *Role Theory and Illness: A Sociological Perspective.* New Haven: Yale University Press.

Gordon, Steve. 1981. "The Sociology of Sentiments and Emotion." In *Social Psychology: Sociological Perspectives.* New York: Basic Books.

Gross, Edward. 1987. "Waiting for Mayo." *Qualitative Sociology* 15:139–164.

Hackett, Thomas P., and Ned H. Cassem. 1979. "Psychological Management of the Myocardial Patient." In *Stress and Survival: The Emotional Realities of Life-Threatening Illness,* ed. Charles A. Garfield, 201–213. St. Louis: Mosby.

Hadden, Stuart C., and Marilyn Lester. 1978. "Talking Identity: The Production of 'Self' in Interaction." *Human Studies* 1:331–356.

Hall, Edward T. 1983. *The Dance of Life.* Garden City, N.Y.: Doubleday.

Hardesty, Carolyn. 1987. "Pain." In *With Wings: An Anthology of Literature by and about Women with Disabilities,* ed. Marsha Saxton and Florence Howe, 19–23. New York: Feminist Press.

Hawking, Stephen W. 1988. *A Brief History of Time.* New York: Bantam.

Hendricks, Jon. 1982. "Time and Social Science." In *Time and Aging,* ed. Ephraim H. Mizruchi, Barry Glassner, and Thomas Pastorello, 12–45. Bayside, N.Y.: General Hall.

Herzlich, C. 1973. *Health and Illness: A Social Psychological Perspective*. London: Academic Press.

Hirsch, Ernest. 1977. *Starting Over*. Hanover, Mass.: Christopher.

Hochschild, Arlie R. 1975. "The Sociology of Feeling and Emotion: Selected Possibilities." In *Another Voice*, ed. Marcia Millman and Rosabeth Moss Kanter, 280–307. Garden City, N.Y.: Anchor Books.

———. 1979. "Emotion Work, Feeling Rules and Social Structure." *American Journal of Sociology* 85:551–575.

———. 1983. *The Managed Heart: Commercialization of Human Feeling*. Berkeley: University of California Press.

Hodgins, Eric. 1964. *Episode: Report on the Accident Inside My Skull*. New York: Atheneum.

Hoffman, Joan Eakin. 1981. "Care of the Unwanted: Stroke Patients in a Canadian Hospital." In *Health and Canadian Society*, ed. David Coburn, Carl D'Arcy, Peter New, and George Torrance, 292–302. Don Mills, Ontario: Fitzhenry & Whiteside Limited.

Hopper, Susan. 1981. "Diabetes as a Stigmatized Condition." *Social Science and Medicine* 15B:11–19.

Idler, Ellen L. 1979. "Definitions of Health and Illness and Medical Sociology." *Social Science and Medicine* 13:723–731.

Izard, C. E. 1977. *Human Emotions*. New York: Plenum.

Jaffe, Lois, and Arthur Jaffe. 1977. "Terminal Candor and the Coda Syndrome: A Tandem View of Fatal Illness." In *New Meanings of Death*, ed. Herman Fiefel, 195–212. New York: McGraw-Hill.

Jaques, Elliott. 1982. *The Form of Time*. New York: Crane Russak.

Jobling, Ray. 1977. "Learning to Live with It: An Account of Dermatological Illness and Patienthood." In *Medical Encounters*, ed. A. Davis and G. Horobin, 72–86. London: Croom Helm.

———. 1988. "The Experience of Psoriasis Under Treatment." In *Living with Chronic Illness*, ed. Robert Anderson and Michael Bury, 224–245. London: Unwin Hyman.

Johnson, Colleen Leahy. 1985. "The Impact of Illness on Late-Life Marriages." *Journal of Marriage and the Family* 47:165–172.

Jones, James M. 1988. "Cultural Differences in Temporal Perspectives: Instrumental and Expressive Behaviors in Time." In *The Social Psychology of Time: New Perspectives*, ed. Joseph E. McGrath, 21–38. Newbury Park, Calif.: Sage.

Jourard, Sidney. 1971. *The Transparent Self*. New York: Van Nostrand.

Karp, David. 1988. "A Decade of Reminders: Changing Age Consciousness Between Fifty and Sixty Years Old." *Gerontologist* 28:727–738.

Katovich, Michael A. 1987. "An Interactionist Approach to the Passage of Time in Film." Paper presented at the Society for the Study of Symbolic Interactionism Gregory P. Stone Symposium, Urbana, Illinois, May 7–9.

Kelleher, David. 1988. "Coming to Terms with Diabetes: Coping Strategies and Non-Compliance." In *Living with Chronic Illness*, ed. Robert Anderson and Michael Bury, 155–187. London: Unwin Hyman.

Kelly, Orville E. 1977. "Make Today Count." In *New Meanings of Death*, ed. Herman Fiefel, 181–194. New York: McGraw-Hill.

Kemper, Theodore D. 1978. *A Social Interactional Theory of Emotions*. New York: John Wiley.

Kestenbaum, Victor. 1982. "The Experience of Illness." In *The Humanity of the Ill*, ed. Victor Kestenbaum, 3–38. Knoxville: University of Tennessee Press.

Kidel, Mark. 1988. "Illness and Meaning." In *The Meaning of Illness*, ed. Mark Kidel and Susan Rowe-Leete, 4–21. London: Routledge.

Kleinman, Arthur. 1988. *The Illness Narratives: Suffering, Healing & the Human Condition*. New York: Basic Books.

Kotarba, Joseph A. 1983. *Chronic Pain: Its Social Dimensions*. Beverly Hills, Calif.: Sage.

Kübler-Ross, Elisabeth. 1969. *On Death and Dying*. New York: Macmillan.

Kutner, Nancy G. 1987. "Social Worlds and Identity in End-Stage Renal Disease (ESRD)." In *Research in the Sociology of Health Care: The Experience and Management of Chronic Illness*, ed. Julius A. Roth and Peter Conrad, 6:33–72. Greenwich, Conn.: JAI Press.

Laird, Carobeth. 1979. *Limbo: A Memoir about Life in a Nursing Home by a Survivor*. Novato, Calif.: Chandler & Sharp.

Lear, Martha Weinman. 1980. *Heartsounds*. New York: Simon & Schuster.

Lee, Laurel. 1987. "Walking through the Fire: A Hospital Journal." In *With Wings: An Anthology of Literature by and about Women with Disabilities*. ed. Marsha Saxton and Florence Howe, 109–115. New York: Feminist Press.

LeMaistre, Joanne. 1985. *Beyond Rage: The Emotional Impact of Chronic Illness*. Oak Park, Ill.: Alpine Guild.

Levinson, Daniel J., C. Darrow, E. Klein, M. Levinson, and B. McKee. 1978. *The Seasons of a Man's Life*. New York: Knopf.

Lewis, Helen Block. 1971. *Shame and Guilt in Neurosis*. New York: International Universities Press.

Lewis, Kathleen. 1985. *Successful Living with Chronic Illness*. Wayne, N.J.: Avery.

Lifton, Robert J. 1968. *Death in Life*. New York: Random House.

Lindesmith, Alfred, Anselm L. Strauss, and Norman K. Denzin. 1975. *Social Psychology*. Hinsdale, Ill.: Dryden Press.

Locker, David. 1981. *Symptoms and Illness: The Cognitive Organization of Disorder*. London: Tavistock.

———. 1983. *Disability and Disadvantage: The Consequences of Chronic Illness*. London: Tavistock.

Lofland, John. 1969. *Deviance and Identity*. Englewood Cliffs, N.J.: Prentice-Hall.

Lofland, John, and Lyn H. Lofland. 1984. *Analyzing Social Settings*. Belmont, Calif.: Wadsworth.

Lofland, Lyn H. 1982. "Loss and Human Connection: An Exploration in the Nature of the Social Bond." In *Personality, Roles and Social Behavior*, ed. William Ickes and Eric S. Knowles, 219–242. New York: Springer-Verlag.

———. 1985. "The Social Shaping of Emotion: The Case of Grief." *Symbolic Interaction* 8:171–190.

Lopata, Helena Znaniecki. 1969. "Loneliness: Forms and Components." *Social Problems* 17:248–262.

———. 1986. "Time in Anticipated Future and Events in Memory." *American Behavioral Scientist* 29:695–709.

Lorber, Judith. 1975. "Good Patients and Problem Patients." *Journal of Health and Social Behavior* 16:213–225.

Lowenberg, June S. 1989. *Caring & Responsibility: The Crossroads Between Holistic Practice and Traditional Medicine.* Philadelphia: University of Pennsylvania Press.

Lynch, Dorothea, and Eugene Richards. 1986. *Exploding into Life.* New York. Aperture.

MacDonald, Lea. 1988. "The Experience of Stigma: Living with Rectal Cancer." In *Living with Chronic Illness,* ed. Robert Anderson and Michael Bury, 177–202. London: Unwin Hyman.

McGrail, Joie Harrison. 1978. *Fighting Back: One Woman's Struggle Against Cancer.* New York: Harper & Row.

McGrath, Joseph E. 1988. "Time and Social Psychology." In *The Social Psychology of Time,* ed. Joseph E. McGrath, 255–267. Beverly Hills, Calif.: Sage.

McGrath, Joseph E., and Janice R. Kelly. 1986. *Time and Human Interaction: Toward a Social Psychology of Time.* New York: Guilford.

McGuire, Meredith B., and Debra J. Kantor. 1987. "Belief Systems and Illness Experience." In *Research in the Sociology of Health Care: The Experience and Management of Chronic Illness,* ed. Julius A. Roth and Peter Conrad, 6: 241–248. Greenwich, Conn.: JAI Press.

McMahan, A. W., and P. J. Rhudick. 1964. "Reminiscing: Adaptational Significance in the Aged." *Archives of General Psychiatry* 10:292–298.

Madruga, Lenor. 1979. *One Step at a Time.* New York: McGraw-Hill.

Maines, David R. 1983. "Time and Biography in Diabetic Experience." *Mid-American Review of Sociology* 8:103–117.

———. 1984. "The Social Arrangements of Diabetic Self-help Groups." In *Chronic Illness and the Quality of Life,* ed. Anselm L. Strauss et al., 111–126. St. Louis: Mosby.

Maines, David R., and Monica J. Hardesty. 1987. "Temporality and Gender: Young Adults' Career and Family Plans." *Social Forces* 66:102–120.

Maines, David R., Noreen M. Sugrue, and Michael A. Katovich. 1983. "The Sociological Import of G. H. Mead's Theory of the Past." *American Sociological Review* 48:161–173.

Mairs, Nancy. 1986. *Plaintext.* Tucson: University of Arizona Press.

Mann, Harriet, Miriam Siegler, and Humphry Osmond. 1972. "The Psychotypology of Time." In *The Future of Time,* ed. Henri Yaker, Humphry Osmond, and Frances Cheek, 142–178. Garden City, N.Y.: Anchor Books.

Mann, Thomas. 1927. *The Magic Mountain.* New York: Knopf.

Marcus, George E., and Michael M. J. Fischer. 1986. *Anthropology as Cultural Critique.* Chicago: University of Chicago Press.

Marris, Peter. 1974. *Loss and Change*. New York: Random House.

Marshall, Victor W. 1980. *Last Chapters: A Sociology of Aging and Dying*. Monterey, Calif.: Brooks-Cole.

Mead, George Herbert. 1932. *The Philosophy of the Present*. LaSalle, Ill.: Open Court.

——. 1934. *Mind, Self and Society*. Chicago: University of Chicago Press.

Melbin, Murray. 1987. *Night as Frontier: Colonizing the World After Dark*. New York: Free Press.

Miall, Charlene E. 1986. "The Stigma of Involuntary Childlessness." *Social Problems* 33:268–283.

Miall, Charlene E., and Nancy Herman. 1986. "Fostering Identities: The Management of Information in 'Normal' and 'Deviant' Worlds." Paper presented at Qualitative Research Conference, University of Waterloo, May 13–16.

Mishler, Elliot G. 1981. "The Social Construction of Illness." In *Social Contexts of Health, Illness & Patient Care*, ed. Elliot G. Mishler, Lorna R. AmaraSingham, Stuart T. Hauser, Ramsay Liem, Samuel D. Osherson, and Nancy Waxler, 141–168. Cambridge, Eng.: Cambridge University Press.

——. 1986. *Research Interviewing: Context and Narrative*. Cambridge: Harvard University Press.

Mitteness, Linda S. 1987. "So What Do You Expect When You're 85?: Urinary Incontinence in Late Life." In *Research in the Sociology of Health Care: The Experience and Management of Chronic Illness*, ed. Julius A. Roth and Peter Conrad, 6:177–220. Greenwich, Conn.: JAI Press.

Morgan, David L. 1982. "Failing Health and the Desire for Independence: Two Conflicting Aspects of Health Care in Old Age." *Social Problems* 30:40–50.

Morgan, John. 1988. "Living with Renal Failure on Home Haemodialysis." In *Living with Chronic Illness*, ed. Robert Anderson and Michael Bury, 203–224. London: Unwin Hyman.

Murphy, Robert F. 1987. *The Body Silent*. New York: Henry Holt.

Nurius, Helen S. 1989. "The Self-Concept: A Social Cognitive Update." *Social Casework* 70:285–294.

Ornstein, Robert E. 1969. *On the Experience of Time*. New York: Penguin Books.

Parsons, Talcott. 1953. *The Social System*. Glencoe, Ill.: Free Press.

Pearlin, Leonard I. 1989. "The Sociological Study of Stress." *Journal of Health and Social Behavior* 30:241–269.

Pearlin, Leonard I., and Carol S. Aneshensel. 1986. "Coping and Social Supports: Their Functions and Applications." In *Applications of Social Science to Clinical Medicine and Health Policy*, ed. Linda H. Aiken and David Mechanic, 417–437. New Brunswick, N.J.: Rutgers University Press.

Petch, M. C. 1983. "Coronary Bypasses." *British Medical Journal* 287:514–516.

Peyrot, Mark, James F. McMurray, Jr., and Richard Hedges. 1987. "Living with Diabetes: The Role of Personal and Professional Knowledge in Symptom and Regimen Management." In *Research in the Sociology of*

Health Care: The Experience and Management of Chronic Illness, ed. Julius A. Roth and Peter Conrad, 6:107–146. Greenwich, Conn.: JAI Press.

———. 1988. "Marital Adjustment to Adult Diabetes: Interpersonal Congruence and Spouse Satisfaction." *Journal of Marriage and the Family* 6:363–376.

Pill, Roisin, and Nigel C. H. Stott. 1982. "Concepts of Illness Causation and Responsibility: Some Preliminary Data from a Sample of Working Class Mothers." *Social Science and Medicine* 16:43–52.

Pinder, Ruth. 1988. "Striking Balances: Living with Parkinson's Disease." In *Living with Chronic Illness*, ed. Robert Anderson and Michael Bury, 67–88. London: Unwin Hyman.

Pitzele, Sefra Kobrin. 1985. *We Are Not Alone: Learning to Live with Chronic Illness*. New York: Workman.

Plough, Alonzo. 1986. *Borrowed Time: Artificial Organs and the Politics of Extending Lives*. Philadelphia: Temple University Press.

Ponse, Barbara. 1976. "Secrecy in the Lesbian World." *Urban Life* 5:313–338.

Quint, Jeanne C. 1965. "Institutionalized Practices of Information Control." *Psychiatry* 28:119–132.

Radley, Alan, and Ruth Green. 1987. "Illness as Adjustment: A Methodology and Conceptual Framework." *Sociology of Health & Illness* 9:179–207.

Radner, Gilda. 1989. *It's Always Something*. New York: Simon & Schuster.

Register, Cheri. 1987. *Living with Chronic Illness*. New York: Free Press.

Reif, Laura. 1975. "Ulcerative Colitis: Strategies for Managing Life." In *Chronic Illness and the Quality of Life*, ed. Anselm L. Strauss and Barney G. Glaser, 81–88. St. Louis: Mosby.

Ressmeyer, Roger. 1983. "A Day to Day Struggle." In *California Living, San Francisco Chronicle & Examiner*. July 10, 1–5.

Revere, V., and S. Tobin. 1980–1981. "Myth and Reality: The Older Person's Relationship to His Past." *International Journal of Aging and Human Development* 12:15–26.

Richardson, Laurel. 1990. "Narrative and Sociology." *Journal of Contemporary Ethnography* 19:116–135.

Robboy, Howard, and Bernard Goldstein. 1987. "Continuous Medical Emergencies and Routinization: Ventilator-Dependent Patients and Their Care-Takers." Trenton State College.

Robinson, David. 1971. *The Process of Becoming Ill*. London: Routledge.

Robinson, Ian. 1988a. "Reconstructing Lives: Negotiating the Meaning of Multiple Sclerosis." In *Living with Chronic Illness*, ed. Robert Anderson and Michael Bury, 43–66. London: Unwin Hyman.

———. 1988b. *Multiple Sclerosis*. London: Tavistock.

Roth, Julius A. 1957. "Ritual and Magic in the Control of Contagion." *American Sociological Review* 22:310–314.

———. 1963. *Timetables*. New York: Bobbs-Merrill.

Ruzek, Sheryl Burt. 1979. *The Women's Health Movement: Feminist Alternatives to Medical Control*. New York: Praeger.

Sacks, Oliver. 1984. *A Leg to Stand On*. New York: Summit Books.

San Francisco Chronicle. 1978. "Looking into the Black Hole of Death." February 8, 13.

Sarton, May. 1988. *After the Stroke: A Journal.* New York: Norton.

Scambler, Graham, and Anthony Hopkins. 1986. "Being Epileptic: Coming to Terms with Stigma." *Sociology of Health & Illness* 8:26–43.

———. 1988. "Accommodating Epilepsy in Families." In *Living with Chronic Illness*, ed. Robert Anderson and Michael Bury, 156–176. London: Unwin Hyman.

Scheff, Thomas J. 1977. "The Distancing of Emotion in Ritual." *Current Anthropology* 18:483–505.

———. 1989. "Toward a Theory of Self-Esteem." Paper presented at the Pacific Sociological Association. Reno, April 13–16.

———. 1990. *Microsociology: Discourse, Emotion, and Social Structure.* Chicago: University of Chicago Press.

Scheler, Max. 1961. *Ressentiment.* Glencoe, Ill.: Free Press.

Schlenker, Barry. 1980. *Impression Management: The Self-Concept, Social Identity and Interpersonal Relations.* Monterey, Calif.: Brooks-Cole.

Schneider, Joseph W., and Peter Conrad. 1980. "In the Closet with Illness: Epilepsy, Stigma Potential, and Information Control." *Social Problems* 28:32–44.

———. 1983. *Having Epilepsy.* Philadelphia: Temple University Press.

Schott, Thomas, and Bernhard Badura. 1988. "Wives of Heart Attack Patients: The Stress of Caring." In *Living with Chronic Illness*, ed. Robert Anderson and Michael Bury, 117–136. London: Unwin Hyman.

Schutz, Alfred. 1971. *Collected Papers.* Vol. 1: *The Problem of Social Reality.* The Hague: Martinus Nijhoff.

Schwartz, Barry. 1975. *Queuing and Waiting: Studies in the Social Organization of Access and Delay.* Chicago: University of Chicago Press.

Schwartz, Susan. 1979. "Cancer Comes Out of the Closet." *Santa Rosa Press Democrat.* September 30, B1–2.

Scott-Maxwell, Florida. 1968. *The Measure of My Days.* New York: Penguin.

Segall, A. 1976. "The Sick Role Concept: Understanding of Illness Behavior." *Journal of Health and Social Behavior* 17:163–170.

Sharron, Avery. 1982. "Dimensions of Time." In *Studies in Symbolic Interaction*, ed. Norman K. Denzin, 4:63–89. Greenwich, Conn.: JAI Press.

Siegler, Miriam, and Humphrey Osmond. 1979. "The 'Sick Role' Revisited." In *Health, Illness and Medicine*, ed. Gary L. Albrecht and Paul C. Higgins, 146–166. Chicago: Rand-McNally.

Simmel, Georg. 1950. *The Sociology of Georg Simmel.* New York: Free Press.

Skevington, Suzanne M. 1986. "Psychological Aspects of Pain in Rheumatoid Arthritis: A Review." *Social Science and Medicine* 23:567–575.

Sontag, Susan. 1978. *Illness as Metaphor.* New York: Farrar, Straus and Giroux.

Sourkes, Barbara M. 1982. *The Deepening Shade.* Pittsburgh: University of Pittsburgh Press.

Speedling, Edward J. 1982. *Heart Attack: The Family Response at Home and in the Hospital.* New York: Tavistock.

Star, Susan Leigh. 1981. "The Social Psychology of Chronic Migraine," Unpublished manuscript, University of California, San Francisco.

———. 1985. "Scientific Work and Uncertainty." *Social Studies of Science* 15:391–427.

Stephens, Joyce. 1976. *Loners, Losers and Lovers.* Seattle: University of Washington Press.

Stewart, David C., and Thomas J. Sullivan. 1982. "Illness Behavior and the Sick Role in Chronic Disease." *Social Science and Medicine* 16:1397–1404.

Stewart, Jean. 1987. "From *The Body's Memory.*" In *With Wings: An Anthology of Literature by and about Women with Disabilities,* ed. Marsha Saxton and Florence Howe, 125–136. New York: Feminist Press.

Strauss, Anselm L. 1964. *George Herbert Mead on Social Psychology.* Chicago: University of Chicago Press.

———. 1969. *Mirrors and Masks.* Mill Valley, Calif.: The Sociology Press.

———. 1987. *Qualitative Analysis for Social Scientists.* Cambridge: Cambridge University Press.

Strauss, Anselm L., and Juliet Corbin. 1984. "Body Failure." Unpublished manuscript, University of California, San Francisco.

———. 1990. *Basics of Qualitative Research: Grounded Theory Procedures and Techniques.* Newbury Park, Calif.: Sage.

Strauss, Anselm L., and Barney G. Glaser. 1975. *Chronic Illness and the Quality of Life* 1st ed. St. Louis: Mosby.

Strauss, Anselm L., Juliet Corbin, Shizuko Fagerhaugh, Barney G. Glaser, David Maines, Barbara Suczek, and Carolyn Wiener. 1984. *Chronic Illness and the Quality of Life.* 2d ed. St. Louis: Mosby.

Strong, Maggie. 1988. *Mainstay.* Boston: Little-Brown.

Sudnow, David. 1967. *Passing On: The Social Organization of Dying.* Englewood Cliffs, N.J.: Prentice-Hall.

Tarman, Vera Ingrid. 1988. "Autobiography." *International Journal of Aging and Human Development* 27:171–191.

Tavris, Carol. 1982. *Anger.* New York: Simon & Schuster.

Taylor, Kathryn M. 1988. "Telling Bad News: Physicians and the Disclosure of Undesirable Information." *Sociology of Health & Illness* 10:109–132.

Telles, Joel Leon, and Mark Harris Pollack. 1981. "Feeling Sick: The Experience and Legitimation of Illness." *Social Science and Medicine* 15:243–251.

Turner, Ralph. 1976. "The Real Self: From Institution to Impulse." *American Journal of Sociology* 81:989–1016.

Turner, Ralph, and Steven Gordon. 1981. "The Boundaries of the Self." In *Self-Concept: Advances in Theory and Research,* ed. Mervin D. Lynch, Ardyth A. Norem-Hebeisen, and Kenneth J. Gergen, 39–73. Cambridge, Mass.: Ballinger.

Twaddle, Andrew C. 1969. "Health Decisions and Sick Role Variations." *Journal of Health and Social Behavior* 10:105–115.

Unruh, David. 1983. "Death and Personal History: Strategies of Identity Preservation." *Social Problems* 30:340–351.

Van den Berg, J. D. 1972, *The Psychology of the Sickbed*. Pittsburgh: Duquesne University Press.

Van Maanen, John. 1988, *Tales of the Field*. Chicago: University of Chicago Press.

Veith, Ilza. 1988. *Can You Hear the Clapping of One Hand?: Learning to Live with a Stroke*. Berkeley, Calif.: University of California Press.

West, Gilly. 1984. "Death Work: An Adjunct to the Hospice Worker, Family, and Patient." Lecture, Gerontology Lecture Series, Sonoma State University, October 25.

Wiener, Carolyn L. 1975. "The Burden of Rheumatoid Arthritis." In *Chronic Illness and the Quality of Life*, Anselm L. Strauss and Barney G. Glaser, 71–80. St. Louis: Mosby.

Williams, Gareth. 1984. "The Genesis of Chronic Illness: Narrative Reconstruction." *Sociology of Health & Illness* 6:175–200.

Williams, R.G.A. 1981a. "Logical Analysis as a Qualitative Method I: Themes in Old Age and Chronic Illness." *Sociology of Health & Illness* 3:140–164.

——. 1981b. "Logical Analysis as a Qualitative Method: Conflict of Ideas and the Topic of Illness." *Sociology of Health & Illness* 3:165–187.

Wilsnack, Richard W. 1980. "Information Control: A Conceptual Framework for Sociological Analysis." *Urban Life* 8:467–500.

Wulf, Helen Harlan. 1979. *Aphasia, My World Alone*. Detroit: Wayne State University Press.

Young, Michael. 1988. *The Metronomic Society: Natural Rhythms and Human Timetables*. Cambridge: Harvard University Press.

Zerubavel, Eviatar. 1979. *Patterns of Time in Hospital Life: A Sociological Perspective*. Chicago: University of Chicago Press.

——. 1981. *Hidden Rhythms: Schedules and Calendars in Social Life*. Chicago: University of Chicago Press.

——. 1982. "Personal Information and Social Life." *Symbolic Interaction* 5:97–109.

Zola, Irving K. 1981. "Structural Constraints in the Doctor-Patient Relationship: The Case of Non-Compliance." In *The Relevance of Social Science for Medicine*, ed. Leon Eisenberg and Arthur Kleinman, 241–252. Reidel: Dordrecht.

——. 1982a. "Introduction." In *Ordinary Lives*, ed. Irving K. Zola, 11–14. Cambridge, Mass.: Apple-wood Books.

——. 1982b. *Missing Pieces: A Chronicle of Living with a Disability*. Philadelphia: Temple University Press.

——. 1986a. "Medicine as an Institution of Social Control." In *The Sociology of Health and Illness*, ed. Peter Conrad and Rochelle Kern, 379–389. New York: St. Martin's.

——. 1986b. "Review of David Locker, *Disability and Disadvantage*." *Qualitative Sociology* 9:92–94.

Zurcher, Louis A. 1982. "The Staging of Emotions: A Dramaturgical Analysis." *Symbolic Interaction* 5:1–27.

Index

acceptance: of death, 246, 247, 249; of illness, 46–49, 65, 244, 281n4; self, 258
accountability for regimen, 157–159
activities: effect of illness, 56, 76; eliminating, 143; in filled present, 241–242; in intense present, 245–250; limiting, 76; past, 193–195; preempted by illness, 57; preserving, 136; reduction, 183, 242; shared, 95; simplifying, 144; in slowed present, 243–245; vital, 58
advocacy, 263, 285n2
anger, 46, 51, 52, 137, 187, 226, 244–245, 251, 254, 282n3
announcements, strategic, 121–127
apnea, 287
appearance: bodily, 70; concern with, 68
assistance. See support
audiences, 36–40, 122; control of, 126
autonomy, 27, 259–260; lack of, 84; loss of, 109–110, 112, 260, 262; maintaining, 131. See also independence
avoidance of disclosure, 110–112, 115–118

bargaining, 48
benefits, disability, 1

carcinoid syndrome, 287
care. See support
cerebral vascular accident, 287
chronic fatigue syndrome, 287–288
chronic illness. See illness
chronicity, 14, 21–23; effect on routines, 21; recovery in, 23; stigma, 22
chronology: collapsed, 237; comparative, 202; of illness, 197–201
colitis, 288
competence, 50, 117
conflicts, time, 154, 171–172
containment of illness, 65–70, 199; packaging, 66–68; passing, 68–70
control, 284n1; of activities, 58; of audiences, 126; bodily, 117; of care, 282n1; challenged, 122; of disclosure, 119; of emotions, 119–121, 127–130, 181; of illness, 44, 57, 212; loss of, 49, 109–110, 185–186, 215–218, 260, 261; of resources, 64; of self, 43; of symptoms, 45, 86, 136; of time, 31, 45, 83
crises, 81; continuing, 185; disruptive, 33–35; identifying, 218; managing, 85–87; start of chronicity, 12; sudden, 28; temporary, 12; time in, 33–35
CVA, 287

days: bad, 49–50, 51–53, 54–56; evaluations, 49–50; existing in, 185–190; good, 3, 41, 49–51; one at a time, 169, 178–185, 239, 243, 283n2; rhythm, 44; routines in, 2, 6–7, 43, 57–58, 82, 237, 249, 283n1; structure, 55
death, 178; acceptance of, 246, 247, 249; awareness of, 14, 99–100, 183; fear of, 98, 125, 156, 179, 251; imminent, 255; threat of, 93

denial, 16–20, 191; definitions, 17; of illness, 16, 20; as label, 17
dependency, 80–81, 102; fear of, 180, 251; physical, 1. *See also* independence
depression, 1, 22, 195, 243, 245, 251, 254
diabetes, 288
diagnosis: and disclosure, 116; evading, 131; lacking, 23–25; meaning, 18; relief at, 24, 57; serious, 28; as timemarker, 202, 203
dialectical self, 70–72
disclosure of illness, 107–133; avoiding, 110–112, 115–118; controlling, 119; planning for, 127–133; problems, 109–110; protective, 119–121; risk in, 112–119; spontaneous, 119–121; staging, 129–130; strategic, 121–127; types, 119–127; and visibility, 111
discoid lupus, 288
disruption, 6, 9, 12; in crises, 33–35; routines, 44; without diagnosis, 23–25
domino effect, 154, 283n6

effects of illness, 21, 56–64, 76, 257–265
emotions: anger, 46, 51, 52, 137, 187, 226, 244–245, 251, 254, 282n3; controlling, 179, 181; fear, 98, 125, 156, 179, 180, 251; grief, 11, 29; guilt, 98, 125; managing, 223; monitoring, 179; negative, 98, 181, 221, 224, 251; past, 218, 223, 224–227; power and, 222; present, 220–224; pride, 166; reliving, 214–220; and self, 220–227; shame, 215, 218, 226, 284n4; shock, 11, 15, 28, 29, 128; transcending, 224–227; unfamiliar, 5
emphysema, 288
events: external, 237; negative, 214–220; positive, 211–214; significant, 207, 210–220, 221, 229
exacerbation of illness, 289
existence, day to day, 185–190

family. *See* relationships
fear, 32; of death, 98, 125, 156, 179, 251; of dependency, 180, 251

friends. *See* relationships
frustration, 51, 52, 137, 244–245
future: assumed, 253–254; contingent, 284n1; dreaded, 33, 235, 250–251; expanded, 170; identity, 101–104; improved, 251–253; planning, 178, 190–193; questionable, 229; role of acceptance, 48; self in, 229, 250–256; uncertain, 32, 178, 180, 235; vague, 35

general assistance, 289
grief, 11, 29
grounded theory method, 273–277
guilt, 98, 125

health care system, 282n1; access to, 264; economics, 2; profit motive, 263; rehabilitation needs, 264; structure, 2, 3, 135. *See also* medical care
Hodgkin's lymphoma, 289
horizons, 96; spatial, 50, 52; temporal, 50, 52
hospice movement, 282n1

iatrogenic effects, 289
identity: appropriate, 48; control of, 45; establishing, 201; future, 101–104; imposed, 102; past, 101–104; preferred, 15; preservation, 255; questioning, 101–104, 219; self, 15, 16, 66, 101–104; social, 15, 151
idiopathic pulmonary fibrosis, 289
illness: acceptance of, 46–49, 65, 244, 281n4; acknowledging, 3, 136, 283n1; acute, 16, 73; chronicity, 14, 21–23; chronology, 197–201; concealing, 69, 110–114; containment of, 5, 65–70, 199; control of, 44, 45, 57, 212; defining, 16, 36, 40, 67; denial of, 16–20; disclosure of, 107–133; effects of, 21, 56–64, 76, 257–265; embracing, 65; environmental, 288–289; episodic, 20, 85–87; flaunting, 126–127; immersion in, 5, 73–104, 189, 199, 207, 235; incorporating, 66, 68; as interruption, 11–40; intrusive, 41–72; living with, 4, 134–166; managing, 57–

58, 82–83, 149, 178, 181; meanings of, 4, 67; onset, sudden, 27–28; packaging of, 66–68; passing with, 68–70; rapid escalation, 23, 25–27; reconciling self to, 47–48; recovery, 12, 13–16; relation to time, 30–35, 88–93, 105, 173, 236, 243, 244, 248; routines, 9, 43, 82–85, 92; social context, 54–55; as temporary condition, 11–12, 30; trajectory, 289

immersion: consequences, 95–104; in crises, 33, 34; in illness, 73–104, 199, 207, 235; in time, 87–93; variations, 93–95

immortality, 255

independence, maintaining, 45, 59, 131, 132, 137, 164, 174, 246. *See also* dependency

Independent Living Movement, 282n1

insurance, 59, 74, 77, 263

interactional: control, 122, 124, 226; risk, 112–113

interruption, illness as, 11–40; defining, 23; recovery, 13–16

intervention, 285n2

intrusion, illness as, 41–72

isolation, 135, 235; reducing, 282n2; social, 82, 95–99, 101, 236

juggling time, 161–166

labeling of denial, 17

life: contexts, 135–137; existing day to day, 185–190; with illness, 4, 134–166; medicalization of, 279n1; one day at a time, 169, 178–185, 239, 243, 283n2; remaking, 76, 138–143; simplifying, 143–152; structure, 58–64

linear temporal world, 284n1

living standards, 145–147

loss, 236, 257–260; of autonomy, 109–110, 112, 260, 262; of control, 31, 49, 109–110, 185, 186, 215–218, 260, 261; in crises, 35; in disclosure, 112–119; past, 240; of self, 221–224, 257, 258, 259; of social contact, 95; and tradeoffs, 151

lupus erythematosus, 289

maintaining: current function, 263–264; independence, 59, 131, 132, 137, 164, 174, 246

managing: crises, 85–87; emotions, 223; illness, 57–58, 82–83, 149, 178, 181; routines, 137–139; self, 178; symptoms, 46; time, 174, 178–190

Medicaid, 2, 279n1, 289–290

medical care: access, 59; compliance, 14–15, 17, 281n4; contradictions, 18; coverage, 59; diagnosis, 18, 23–24; escalation, 38; expectations, 30; lack of control, 217; noncompliance, 137; planning, 17; raising hopes, 19; rejection, 262; role models in, 175–178; system, 261–265

Medicare, 263, 290

medication, side effects, 56, 57

mixed connective tissue disease, 290

monitoring emotions, 179

multiple sclerosis, 290

myasthenia gravis, 290

normalization, 28, 53, 150

observers, 36–40, 122, 126

organization, 138–143

pacing time, 161–166

passivity, 257

past: activities, 193–195; emotions, 218, 223, 224–227; examining, 220; familiar, 233–234; functioning, 22; identity, 87, 101–104; losses, 240; recapturing, 193–195; reconstructed, 234–239; resuming, 33; self, 6, 92, 220–224, 231–239; tangled, 231–233

peripheral neuropathy, 290

perspectives, time, 13, 75, 93–95, 169–195, 283n1

photodermatitis, 290

physicians. *See* medical care

planning: disclosure, 127–133; future, 190–193; medical care, 17

policy, social, 257

power, role in emotions, 222

premature ventricular contraction, 290–291

present: alien, 233–234; dreaded, 34; emotions, 220–224; endless, 62; filled, 241–242; functioning, 22; improbable, 31; intense, 242, 245–250; overwhelming, 86; relating to, 170; self, 51, 101, 127, 210, 220, 237, 239–250; slowed, 243–245; temporary, 149; unsettled, 33, 35
priorities, changing, 14
prognosis, disclosure, 131
protective disclosure, 119–127
public assistance, 289
pursuits. *See* activities
PVC, 290–291

Raynaud's phenomena, 291
reconstructing life, 76, 138–143
recovery, 12, 13–16, 30, 246; in chronicity, 23; meriting, 15; timeout for, 14
regimen, 46, 51, 73. abandoning, 115, 156, 157; changing, 159; contradicting, 134–135; focus on, 178; managing, 137–139, 158; as refuge, 281n3. *See also* routines
rejection, 108, 109
relationships: abandonment, 125; changing, 63–64, 95, 97, 99; conflict in, 149–150; and dependency, 80; and disclosure, 116–117, 130; ethics, 2; expectations, 53; family, 60, 62, 96, 98, 137, 187; lack of control, 217; maintaining, 143; measuring, 123; preserving, 131, 182; problems, 12, 126; pulling in, 81–82; ranking, 82; role in illness, 36–40, 56; and self-concept, 230; strained, 109, 132; tenuous, 114
relief, 35, 57
remission, 291
risk: in disclosure, 112–119; emotional, 121; health, 241; interactional, 112–113; and rejection, 108
role models, 175–178
routines: accountable, 157–159; chronicity effect, 21; daily, 2, 6–7, 43, 57–58, 82, 237, 249, 283n1; illness, 9, 43, 82–85, 92; managing, 137–139; simplified, 143–152; structured, 153

schedules: controlling, 163; time, 152–161
self: altered views, 229, 233; boundaries, 84; concept, 75, 79, 118, 260, 279n2, 280n2; constructing, 4; creation, 84; dialectical, 70–72; diminished, 137, 218, 238; effects of illness, 257–265; esteem, 224; evaluation, 50; expectations, changed, 21, 245; exposure, 121; future, 250–256; identification, 15, 16, 66, 101–104; image, 57, 124, 210, 279n2; limits, 49; loss of, 221–224, 257, 258, 259; measurement, 206; monitoring, 70–72; past, 6, 92, 220–224, 231–239; preferred, 118, 238, 251; present, 51, 101, 127, 210, 220, 237, 239–250; presentation, 66, 68; preservation, 70, 123, 153; private, 66, 116, 223; public, 66; real, 15, 194, 221, 229, 230, 247, 280n2; redefining, 227; respect, 260; retreating into, 100; retrieving a past, 14, 21–23, 190, 193–195; revealing, 108; in time, 228–256; transcendence of, 224, 257–260; transformed, 201; worth, 45
shame, 215, 218, 226, 284n4
shock, 11, 15, 28, 29, 128
"sick role," 13
Sjögren's syndrome, 291
social: contact, 96, 97; context of illness, 54–55; horizons, 96; identity, 15, 151; isolation, 82, 95–99, 101, 236; policy, 257; restrictions, 84; support, 59, 158, 254
Social Security, 1, 2
spontaneous disclosure, 119–127
SSI, 2, 187, 291
standards of living, 145–147
stereotypes, 48
stigmatization, 2, 22, 27, 49–50, 66, 109, 110, 112, 113, 117, 258
strategies: living with illness, 134–166
stress, 23
Supplemental Security Income, 2, 187, 291
support, 46; attendant, 74, 84, 150, 165–166; commitments, 125; eco-

nomic, 59; family, 60, 62, 96, 137, 187; financial, 61–62, 77, 78; lack of, 81, 185; in managing, 82, 141; professional, 128–129; social, 59, 254

symbols of illness, 27

symptoms, 32; control of, 45, 86; devastating, 82; discounting, 40; experiencing, 29; ignoring, 49; intrusive, 44–45; invisible, 56–57; management of, 46; normalization, 28; recurrent, 24; undiagnosed, 31–32; vague, 23, 25, 205; visible, 57

systemic lupus erythematosus, 289

telling. *See* disclosure of illness

temporal incongruence, 171–175

testing, 28–29

time: altered, 171–195, 210; bad days, 49–50, 51–53; buffer, 33; changes, 4–5; chronology, 198–201; conflicts, 154, 171–172; control of, 31, 45, 83; crisis, 33–35; dragging, 90–91; drifting, 90–91; duration, 88–93, 105, 173, 236, 243, 244, 248; elusive, 29–30; experiencing, 4, 29–35, 93; filling, 187–188; good days, 49–51; horizons, 239; immersion, 87–93; juggling, 161–166; managing, 174, 178–190; movement of, 280n7; neutral, 282n4; pacing, 161–166; perspectives, 13, 75, 93–95, 169–195, 283n1; reordering, 152–161, 248; in retrospect, 91–92; scheduling, 152–161; self in, 228–256; structures, 169–195; temporal incongruence, 171–175; unchanging, 87–90, 236, 282n5; using, 3; waiting, 30–33

timeframes, 62, 154; self in, 229

timemarkers, 6, 177, 196–197, 260; diagnosis as, 202, 203; establishing, 201–207; identifying moments, 207–210; illness, 198–207; as measures, 206–207; social consequences, 203–204

timeout, 172; for recovery, 14, 177; for rest, 155

tradeoffs, 162, 283n3; simplifying life, 143–152; time scheduling, 152–161

transcendence, 224–227, 257–260

trust, 223

turning points, 6, 210–220, 221, 229, 258, 260

validation: of illness, 24–25, 28; of past self, 235, 238

victimization, 38, 79

vulnerability, 189

worth, diminished, 2

Printed in the United States
2478

9 780813 519678